The Lantern of Tai Chi

Lighting the Path Ahead for an Ancient Art

Brian L. Meyers

Edited by Francesca Amendolia

Printed in the United States of America

First Printing, 2024

ISBN 978-1-955791-36-6

Library of Congress Control Number: Pending

Ordering Information: Special discounts are available on quantity purchases by bookstores, corporations, associations, and others. For details, contact the publisher at sales@braughlerbooks.com or at 937-58-BOOKS.

For questions or comments about this book, please write to info@braughlerbooks.com.

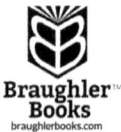

Braughler™
Books
braughlerbooks.com

Acknowledgements

Tim Coletta, my teacher. He is senior master teacher of Kempo, Jeet Kun Do and Tai Chi Chuan. This book would clearly not be possible without him.

My teachers Jenn McWilliams and Mike Stevens, who have contributed greatly to my understanding, practice, and skill.

Yap Boh Heung, master of the Southern Shaolin internal art of WuMei and Yan Shou Gong Qi Gong. I am especially grateful for his "Road Map" of internal martial arts.

Tony Taylor, student of Yi Chuan, who tried so patiently to teach me the 108-Step Form.

My friends and colleagues in the Cincinnati Tai Chi community

Neil B. Anderson, licensed massage therapist and student of the internal arts. The Fabric Model of the body came from him.

Readers: Dr. Linda Davis, Brad Ostendorf, and Deb Wang.

My friends at Parkinson Community Fitness

Francesca Amendolia, editor

Dedications

My love of the art and all of the wisdom contained in these pages came from my teachers and mentors. I am grateful to them for all of it.

All of the details came from my research. Any mistakes and inaccuracies are my own.

This book is dedicated to Alayna – Fare forward, Voyager.

And with profound thanks to my family and my friends.

Table of Contents

Introduction

Sometimes, when I think about Tai Chi, I am reminded of my hero "Number 10 Ox." He is the legendary adventurer and detective's assistant who played a crucial role in solving the mystery of *The Bridge of Birds*, a fantasy romance novel about legendary China written by Barry Hughart. My affection for Number 10 Ox may relate to my place in class or to the grace with which I move through my forms. For my part, I am honored to play the role of detective's assistant in exploring and explaining the esoteric and more prosaic mysteries of Tai Chi Chuan, Grand Ultimate Fist—or, as it is more commonly called, Tai Chi. It seems to be a common narrative structure that the assistant is called upon to do the humble work of telling the story while the master detective (a.k.a. my teacher) does the heavy lifting of deciphering and teaching the mysteries of the Cosmos.

While there are many, many books about Tai Chi and I have enjoyed reading many of them, my hope is this one is a little different. This book is intended to introduce Tai Chi to readers and students who are interested in the art and want to learn more about it. An additional goal is to offer descriptions of the lore, basic concepts, and core principles in a manner that is thought and conversation provoking. This book may be whimsical at moments. It may be amusing, and it might even be—dare I hope—interesting. However, it is also the result of careful study, meticulous practice, and a lot of work. It has been said that Tai Chi represents a journey of personal development. It has also been called the science of self-awareness. But be warned: If you fall in love with the art, as I and my colleagues have, it will captivate your imagination for the rest of your life

1

and influence how you move through your day. Thank you for that affliction, my Teacher.

You may recall that old story about some blind fools who encountered an elephant for the first time. Each was asked to describe what he found; his impression of the animal. One man found the trunk and described an enormous boa constrictor. One man found the elephant's leg and described a sturdy tree trunk. One man felt the elephant's flank and compared the rough skin to a wall. One man grabbed hold of the elephant's tail and compared the animal to a rope. According to the story, these blind fools spent the remainder of the afternoon arguing about who was right and who was describing the elephant properly. Actually, all of those fools were right in part— and they were all wrong. They were each describing their individual experiences. The problem is their experiences of the elephant were piecemeal, objectivist, reductionist, and hardly wholistic. Their descriptions had the effect of breaking the poor animal into distinct pieces. In essence, they butchered it. The description of Tai Chi that you will find in this book also includes descriptions of many disparate pieces; however, as we will see, each piece is in fact a thread of a whole fabric with many and varied designs.

Describing Tai Chi is every bit like describing an encounter with an elephant. There are many aspects, a variety of moving parts, and many levels of understanding. Happily for you, my dear reader, I am eager to describe as many parts of Tai Chi as I can get my hands on, so to speak: the trunk, tail, skin, and legs, and everything in between.

Continuing the comparison of elephants to Tai Chi, my teacher is the true elephant handler. He is familiar with all of the disparate parts. He also has an intuitive understanding of the elephant's personality, its intelligence, and how to care for it so that it grows and prospers. He has an intuitive grasp that the whole of the animal is far greater than the description of its parts. So while I will present it here piece by piece, I hope we can eventually reassemble all of the parts into a useful whole.

Having said all of that, you will find in these pages all the discussions one might expect from a book about Tai Chi: what it is, where it came from, how to learn it, etc. It includes the important bits students should know (those my teacher has sought to impress upon me). Other parts are more introspective—creative, amusing, and possibly hyperbolic. This book also represents the distillation of notes I've made from years of class experiences, discussions with my teachers and colleagues, research, and explorations.

One advantage I have in telling the story of Tai Chi is that I am not too far removed from feeling self-conscious and foolish about my own practice.[1] Yes, Besotted Monkey Tai Chi is a real thing, and I'll tell you about that later. I have practiced every day for years, and my teacher still scolds me about my posture, the empty step, or about moving more quietly. I remember what it's like to be a student and what it's like trying to explain Tai Chi to someone who has never done it. And that is exactly what this book is all about.

In today's world, we have better, more complex, and more precise language to use in describing what might be difficult concepts. However, sometimes the language of clear explanation is difficult to find. In the following pages, I have drawn on stories, anecdotes, and metaphors that walk the line between being common enough to be clear in their meaning and specific enough to inspire novel thinking and discussion. Also, in order to explain the ideas of the art, I have drawn heavily on the language of mental health, the uplifting perspective of professional coaching, and philosophical inquiry. In essence, the language and ideas I've used to describe the art of Tai Chi are updated for contemporary readers. At the same time, I have sought to present an authentic description that is respectful of traditional teachings.

Nevertheless, if you are looking for a book written by a master, that is not me. I am not a master, not even close, and so this might

---

1   There are plenty of days when I feel very confident about my practice. Even better, there are many days when I just practice. I don't "think" about it at all. We will talk about that later.

not be your book. Maybe you should put it down now. Go ahead. Put it down now before you get sucked in.

On the other hand, if you are looking for a book about Tai Chi written by someone who is passionate about the art, who still feels compelled to prove his worth by meticulously doing his homework, who is interested in better understanding the art and how to teach it, and who is pretty darn cheeky when it comes to telling a good story, you'll enjoy this.

The Lantern of Tai Chi

While I write this at Starbucks, a man over there is evidently practicing his imaginary golf swing. He's leaning over, eyeing his imaginary tee'd-up ball, and turning his hips to bring his imaginary club around. It looks like he is trying to stretch out his shoulders and back.

I want to tell him about a Qi Gong exercise for improving one's golf swing. I want to tell him to stand up straight, gently twist the shoulders contra to the hips, and feel the play of the core muscles as he moves. Twist the spine, but don't tense the muscles. Instead, relax and be gentle, and don't twist farther than needed. There is no need to strain, reach too far, or stress out. Activate the abs (the oblique abdominus and transvers abdominus muscles that girdle the core and help us to turn and twist). I want to tell him to imagine sending energy through them but without tensing or pushing too far. The activation of muscles does not require resistance. Yes, there are times when resistance training, weights, and so on are useful to build muscles. This is not one of those times. Here, you want to feel the muscles but relax. Using the muscles intentionally increases blood and energy flow through them. Essentially, moving works out the kinks.

The question is this: How would I explain Qi Gong in ten seconds or less to a man who quite likely has no idea what it is? And what the blazes is Qi Gong, anyway? Now that I've finished writing, I guess could just say, "Here! Read this book." And if I ever see that guy again, maybe I will.

Me? I have been a student of Tai Chi for more than 10 years, a traveler along the path. Sometimes, I am a journeyman instructor. I taught people with Parkinson's disease at a neighborhood resource center, Parkinson Community Fitness. I have learned so much from my students there, and I'm grateful. I am also fortunate to have a phenomenal teacher who guides me in my efforts. I have a background in yoga and have spent time studying other martial arts.

A word about yoga and other martial arts—I have a 200-hour teaching certification in Yin or Daoist yoga. I rely on this experience to help explain body structure in general and muscular and myofascial structure in particular. I also hold belt ranks in Shotokan karate, Aikido, Krav Maga, and Kempo. As you can see, I have my own experiences exploring various movement and martial arts styles. All of this helps me to understand and explain how the Qi energy system works. In fact, all the various martial arts I've studied help me to better understand Tai Chi by contrast.

Also, I would really like to tell you a little bit about my teacher. If anyone should be considered a master, it is him—although I have never heard him accept the accolade or the burden of that title. He has more than five decades of study, an engineer's sense of problem solving, and a deeply intuitive grasp of the martial arts. He is always eager to explore the mysteries of the Cosmos and he is very much at home in the woods. In addition, he counts among his own teachers some of the greatest names in the martial arts community of his generation.

In no small bit of irony for today's world, he is also very humble. He is not the sort of man who wishes to seek the spotlight. You won't find him on YouTube or TikTok. He is more interested in seeking greater understanding than in seeking fame. So for the purposes of this book, I will refer to him as simply Sifu, my teacher.

Then, there's this: Tai Chi comprises a body of information, wisdom, lore, and principles. All of that represents the traditions of Tai Chi. Without all of that, we wouldn't have an art that is true to its historical nature or character. Those traditions represent a cohesive body of wisdom that can be passed from one generation to the next. How does that work? How do those traditions get transmitted from one generation to the next and maintain their cohesion and integrity? How do we pass it along without eroding the message? How do we keep that message from getting garbled or losing its power as it gets handed down from one generation to the next? How do we light the way forward for the generations that come after us?

Tai Chi finds its roots in ancient China. Metaphorically, metaphysically, and philosophically speaking, the art is an alloy or melding of what might arguably be described as the teachings of ancient Chinese Buddhist and Daoist psycho-somatic mystery schools. That just means they were interested in exploring the mysteries of connecting and coordinating the body, mind, spirit. The art was later burnished by Confucian thinkers interested in community and society building. Tai Chi is forged in the physical, psychological, and spiritual crucibles of the Buddhist monks who sought physical conditioning to reinforce their prayer and meditation practices and by the Daoist mountain men who hammered the steel of the art in the cold, early mornings before their grass huts or mountain caves. It is easy to imagine that both monks and mountain men began by trying to stretch out the stiff kinks and aches from a night's slumbers. Maybe they were trying to reclaim the lost energy and vitality of youth. Maybe they wanted to capture the romantic idylls of mysticism or slough off the drowsy hangovers of long hours of prayer or meditation (or even possibly the concoctions and distillations of gathered plants). Maybe, they wanted to tease out the secrets of life and its inevitable conclusion. We might suggest that all of them fancied themselves alchemists, mystics, immortals, or madmen. The stories about their efforts likely wrote themselves, and maybe the stories are true.

And while we will get into this later in the book, let me say two things. First, the stretching out of kinks and reclaiming our vitality are all natural impulses of the human condition. All humans get old and stiff and sore. At least, the lucky among us do. We all have an instinct to stave off or avoid life's inevitable conclusion.

Second, humans also have an instinct to explore and commune with the mysteries of the Cosmos, however we may describe them. We seek meaning for our lives. These human impulses are common to everyone. These early Buddhist monks and Daoist mountain men took those impulses and made them into an early science that unifies the body, mind, and spirit. That science has been gathering information and understanding for many centuries. Later on Chinese imperials got a hold of the art, and much like the imperial dynasties that preceded them, the Red Dynasty in particular sought to capture the art, refine it, and harness it to help create a great society. Even after revolutions and Great Leaps Forward, the Chinese have never seemed to wander far from the power of their Confucian roots. All of this smelting, hammering, and refining formed the traditions and lore of Tai Chi. And that, my friend, is the elephant in the room.

But there have been innovators along the way, too. We want to talk about the relationships between the traditions and the innovators and artists. Without those storied traditions, wisdom, and lore, Tai Chi would be formless and void of meaning. There would be no message; nothing to transmit across the ages. It would have no power to speak to current and future generations. Then, we think about the artists in every generation who pushed the boundaries of understanding. Without the innovators and artists who add exploration and self-expression, the art would never grow. It would become stale and stagnant. Its language would become archaic and dismissed as a relic of history. But Tai Chi as a body of knowledge and understanding is every bit as vibrant, vigorous, and relevant today as it has ever been. In fact, in today's language, we might even refer to it as "tech for hacking the mind and body."

When it all comes down to it, there are at least two great ultimate questions about Tai Chi that we need to explore (although there are many smaller questions we will discuss in coming pages). The first is this: regarding the traditions, lore, and wisdom of Tai Chi and the impermanence of each generation, how do we transmit all these treasures to future generations? How do we light the way ahead for the students currently on their own journeys and those who are yet to come? How do we peer ahead into the darkness of the future? How do we light the lantern? Ultimately, that's what this book is all about.

The second great ultimate question was asked by Scott M. Rodell in his book A Notebook for Students of Tai Chi. With respect, his question is a little more prosaic, a little more ordinary, a little less abstract, and every bit as profound. And we will get to that later too.

Chapter 1: What Is Tai Chi?

Tai Chi, which is shorthand for Tai Chi Chuan[2] or "Grand Ultimate Fist", is a traditional Chinese exercise system. It is widely regarded as both a martial art and a regimen for health and wellbeing. It is best known for its graceful, stylized movements. Tai Chi is practiced very slowly. Every move is intentional and precise. Indeed, people often think of Tai Chi as that exercise that old people do in the park on Saturday mornings. In many respects, that is a well-deserved reputation.

Many people think of Tai Chi as an adjunct health and wellness regimen designed to ward off the ravages of age and dis-ease. That is because many of the activities commonly associated with Tai Chi involve stretching and strengthening muscles and tendons, enhancing mind-body coordination, restoring functional balance, and activating cognitive functioning. All of that just means sloughing off the aches and stiffness and making us use our minds in order to hone our eye-hand coordination, remember the sequence of moves, and learn to move through them without thinking.

Tai Chi can be described as a system for the development of psychosomatic coordination, or mind-body connection. In other words, Tai Chi wants to teach the practitioner how to organize and coordinate their body, internal energy, mind, and spirit. By organizing each of these into a common purpose, we can develop a whole person who is greater than the sum of these parts.

---

2   There are a variety of ways to spell and style the transliterated Tai Chi and Tai Chi Ch'uan—capitalized or not, with apostrophes or not. I am choosing to spell them as Tai Chi and Tai Chi Chuan throughout except (of course) when I am quoting from an author who adhered to a different spelling.

On a deeper level, however, Tai Chi, as an activity, is designed to help us understand, cultivate, and circulate Qi, or life energy, throughout the body. The unbroken circulation of Qi is considered to be a hallmark of good health. Learning to sense and manipulate one's own Qi is one thing. Tai Chi also wants to teach us to understand and manipulate Qi in others, as agents of either healing or harm.

Tai Chi as Martial Art

I would like to spend a moment to talk about self-defense and martial arts. To be sure, these might be obvious in their meaning. But let's dig into them just a bit. First, you should know that Tai Chi does not enjoy a good reputation as a practical martial art. It often requires many years to master, and it requires mastery of oneself before learning to master others. Second, Tai Chi is often compared to other martial arts — boxing for example. Boxers might say that Tai Chi players are not as good at boxing as boxers. And they are exactly right. And every practitioner of any martial art will tell you the same thing. They will assert that their art is the greatest one. However, there are some who assert that Tai Chi is the mother of all martial arts. They mean to suggest that it is the greatest of them all. Having said that, if you want to be a good boxer, then by all means study boxing. It is a fantastic sport, and it has a lot to offer. It is also worth saying that boxers don't often understand Tai Chi. The point is that Tai Chi offers strategies and tools that are different from other martial arts. It offers a robust collection of moves, strikes, defenses, and other functions. It is a powerful study of self-defense. It prefers to deploy strikes from very close range that are intended to disrupt the opponent's structure, balance, and Qi flow. It also wants to teach us how to defend ourselves by maintaining our own physical, mental and spiritual balance. It relies on calm, precise movements and prefers to power those moves by use of coordinated body mechanics and one's own Qi energy instead of relying on athleticism or muscles.

Every move in Tai Chi has apparent and hidden self-defense, martial arts applications, and they are important to understand. At the same time, remember this: Self defense can also mean avoiding or minimizing the effect of a fall on a slippery stair or sidewalk. It could mean learning to manage an emotional or mental health disorder or a movement disorder such as the shuffling gait characteristic of Parkinson's disease. Self-defense might mean supporting a friend who is unsteady or falling. Self-defense can also mean understanding situational awareness. It can help you learn to identify, anticipate, and avoid elements in your environment before they become acutely dangerous.

There is an additional consideration. Many of the historical masters of Tai Chi had good reasons to disguise the martial nature of the art from whatever imperial Chinese government held power. We will also see that the imperial Chinese government had political reasons to strip out the obvious martial nature of the art it sought to teach. So while many people who practice Tai Chi have no interest in learning how to fight, I share my teacher's opinion that understanding Tai Chi as a martial art and understanding the martial applications will help you to better understand Tai Chi and how it works. Many of the conversations in this book take that perspective.

Ultimately, the aim of Tai Chi is to learn to move efficiently without thinking or hesitation and with total calmness. Through Tai Chi, we want to learn to move with the greatest effect to achieve our purpose and expend the least amount of effort or energy possible. We want to learn to make best mechanical use of our bones, muscles, and connective tissue. This is called biomechanical advantage. At the same time, we want to protect our balance and calm our mind and our body. Is this not part of self-defense?

Internal Martial Arts versus External

From a Chinese perspective, the world of martial arts is divided into "internal" styles and "external" ones. Tai Chi is considered an internal or soft martial art. Other examples of internal arts include Tai Chi's sister styles: Bagua Chuan, Xing Yi Chuan, and others.

There is also the Japanese martial art Aikido, which is considered a soft art as well.

Internal arts aim to develop understanding and cultivation of five separate types of energy related to the self in a wholistic sense. The first relates to the physical body: external muscles and also posture and body structure. This is where all students of Tai Chi begin — learning to move their body in an organized, coordinated fashion so that the disparate parts work in conjunction and to common purpose for biomechanical advantage. Even so, we should note that there is not the same emphasis on muscular strength and athleticism as in the external arts. The second level is the mind. This relates to consciousness, awareness, and intellect. However, within the language of traditional Tai Chi, mind most often corresponds to intention. The third level is Qi or internal energy.[3] This is life energy. It represents the fuel source that drives various bodily functions. We can learn to feel Qi, cultivate it and manipulate it. The fourth level is Jin (or Jing). Jin represents the physical expression of Qi energy. Fifth and finally, we have Shen, commonly referred to as spirit. Jin and Shen represent the most esoteric levels of Tai Chi. Of course, we will come back to all of these later. Students of Tai Chi learn that soft can overcome strength and hardness, but unless they come to believe this completely, they are missing the point.

External martial arts, or hard styles, by comparison, include Kung Fu, Karate, Kempo, Krav Maga, boxing, and so on. These arts develop physical strength and athletic ability. These arts value direct confrontation and use of overwhelming physical force to move ahead. External martial arts can be extremely effective for the purposes of combat or self-defense. They can often be learned quite a lot faster than their internal counterparts. They can also be effective for developing a person's character. On the other hand, they can also

3   Qi energy can also be spelled Chi. In Japanese martial arts like Aikido, it is spelled Ki. Also, I want to point out that the word Chi in Tai Chi is a homonym for Qi energy, but it is a different word. Tai Chi Chuan translates as "great ultimate fist," the martial art. For clarity, I'll use Tai Chi to refer to the art Tai Chi Chuan. I'll use Qi to refer to the energy and Taiji, the Great Ultimate, to refer to matters related to cosmology.

put quite a lot of stress and damage on the body. Younger folks who like to fight or who are interested in self-defense often prefer the hard styles. Typically, they have less patience for slow, soft styles. On the other hand, older folks tend to prefer the soft styles because they have a nuanced view of patience and because they take longer to heal from the stress and damage of the external styles.

Kung Fu

Kung Fu, alternatively spelled Gong Fu, is an umbrella term for traditional Chinese martial arts. Kung Fu began and was formalized by Chinese monks in the Shaolin Temple in China over the centuries. They are external or hard arts, and they were originally referred to as Wushu. The term Kung Fu came into common usage when it began to arrive on Western shores in the 1960s and 70s and appear on movie screens. Kung Fu is often associated by proximity with Tai Chi. Many schools today that teach one, offer both. There are thousands of variations of Kung Fu that have developed across China. We will examine a little bit of its history in the next chapter.

Another meaning of Kung Fu

For the purposes of our discussion, however, I offer another meaning of Kung Fu, or Gong Fu. Kung Fu can also refer to any endeavor that requires effort, patience, practice, and presence of mind, something that requires devotion and care. So, for example, sweeping the street can be menial labor if it is done carelessly or sloppily, if it is "just a job." Or if care is taken to do it well and proudly, if an effort is made to find meaning in doing a good job, it can be Kung Fu. Kung Fu can be any endevor in which you are fully present and focused. Learning an art such as Tai Chi (or any other discipline) can be cursory, quickly skimmed over, or approached with half a mind or while distracted. You can look for shortcuts for how to complete the learning quickly. Or you can study with vigor and mindfulness. That is Kung Fu. Internal energy cultivation only comes with patient, careful, dedicated practice of your art. As mentioned, the internal arts focus on this. In a sense, you need the discipline of Kung Fu in order to achieve energy cultivation.

A Few Thoughts

There are a few initial thoughts about Tai Chi that I wish to share:

FIRST: THERE IS NO SINGLE VERSION OF TAI CHI.

There is no monolithic governing body for Tai Chi. Given what I said in the introduction about the traditions of Tai Chi, this might seem contradictory. Sure, there are still "official" families in China such as the Yang, Chen, and Wu families that oversee their own brands of Tai Chi. These go back many generations, as we will see. I'm sure that somewhere in Beijing, there is still a National Athletic Committee that claims authority over all Tai Chi inside the People's Republic of China. Outside of China, these families and organizations hold considerably less authority. The reality is that Tai Chi is in the people's hands now. It is vaguely subversive in the sense that Tai Chi is completely available to anyone. Once you learn it, no one can take it away from you. Once you gain the skills, they are yours for the keeping.

On the other hand, anyone can claim to be a teacher, sifu, master, or what-have-you. There are accreditation organizations such as the American Tai Chi and Qi Gong Association. They base accreditation for teachers, for example, on self-reported hours of practice and teaching and on acquiring letters of reference. While they seem legitimate at a glance, I am not currently associated with them, and I do not have an opinion about their organization. There are also places where you can spend a weekend and become a "master" of Tai Chi. Or during that same weekend, if you spend a little extra money, you can get "certified" to become a teacher. Take these for what they are worth. Any Tai Chi certification, rank, or teaching qualification is only as good as your teacher's reputation and understanding — or as good as the students you teach. How much time do they put in?

How much time do you put in? Sifu often says that if you want to see how good a teacher is, look at their students.

Tai Chi has very little to do with how much money you spend. It has very little to do with achievement either. Instead, it has almost everything to do with how much time, discipline, intention, and intellect you put into it. It represents the study of internal resilience and response to adversity. Once learned, it is yours. No person can take it away from you. Only time and mortality can do that.

SECOND: DON'T WORRY ABOUT BEING GOOD AT TAI CHI

Something else: In the western world, we often judge ourself by how "good" we are at something. With respect to Tai Chi, there really is no being good at it. There is only practice. Let me say that again: There really is no being "good" at it. There is only getting better. There is only practice and improvement. Your teacher will guide you and help you polish your form. And you progress by developing greater understanding as you go. Then one day, you will catch yourself moving differently than you remember. Maybe your posture is different. Maybe you realize that your stiffness has gone away. Maybe you find yourself responding to a stressor or trigger more calmly. These are the markers of progress in Tai Chi.

However, if you train completely on your own, you will quickly run into the limits of your understanding. There is only so far you can go by yourself. You won't have any idea of what more there is to learn, and so you will miss out on a whole lot. There is an absolute benefit to finding the best teacher you can. Happily, there are still great teachers. There is great work in furthering the understanding of the art done in unlikely places. You might be surprised at what you can find in your own neighborhood. This raises an important question: How do you know if you have found a good teacher? We'll look at that, too, in a later chapter.

THIRD: THERE IS NO MIRACLE OR MAGIC TO TAI CHI

A third consideration, and perhaps one more central to our discussion, and it may be a disappointment: There is no miracle to Tai Chi. There is no waving a magic wand or stick or staff or sword that will instantly reveal the mysteries and bestow lifelong benefits. There are no short cuts. There is no immediate gratification. Few teachers offer ranks or belts to mark your progress. To be sure, Tai Chi can do a whole lot for a person, but those benefits are directly correlated to the amount of time and practice you put in. That is why Tai Chi is a journey of no destination. It is almost entirely internally motivated. You must choose for yourself how far you want to take it and how diligently you want to practice. If you allow it, it will become a lifelong pursuit. If you allow it, it will teach you many mysteries. "Enjoy the journey," Sifu has told me many times.

Tai Chi has quite a lot to offer in terms of health benefits. However, it should also be noted that it is not a cure-all. It does not represent an 11-hour absolution for an otherwise poor lifestyle or for those who do not take care of themselves. It is not a good idea, for example, to rely on a Tai Chi practice to compensate for poor dietary habits or poor sleep hygiene. Although, Tai Chi practice is good at helping one become aware of these problems. Still, it would not be a good idea to replace the advice and care of medical and mental health professionals with reliance on a Tai Chi practice. Put another way, the best course of action is to both listen to your doctor and practice Tai Chi.

It's important to note that Tai Chi is for anyone, but it's not for everyone. In other words, Tai Chi is accessible for anyone who can stand, balance on one foot, move, and for anyone who is capable of learning something new. We can even modify the forms to accommodate people who are less abled or who have physical challenges. There is even considerable benefit for people who are chair bound learning to practice the art. They will miss quite a lot — movement, balance and so on — but they can also benefit from moving as well as they can and from studying energetic flow.

However, many folks won't have the patience to continue Tai Chi for long. Some folks like to dabble or see what it's all about, and that is enough for them. That's OK. Tai Chi can be an interesting exploration that lasts an afternoon or an evening. If that's you, be assured that your take-home will be a relaxing, enjoyable experience. That is, if you don't mind beginner's self-consciousness. It can be confusing trying to figure out how to follow along with the others in class. For some folks, the Tai Chi journey is very short. It simply is not their thing. There is nothing wrong with that. For other folks, Tai Chi might become just another exercise class. Maybe they run or lift weights, and they go to Tai Chi class every week. If all they do is go to class a couple of times per week, they will get as far as they get. Maybe they will learn a form or two, but without practice, the forms are quickly forgotten after they stop attending.

For yet other folks, perhaps a very few, every step forward leads to a deepening of their commitment to step forward once again. Keep going. As my teacher says, you will have some great surprises waiting for you.

A common recommendation for people who want to try Tai Chi is to give it at least three months to decide if you like it. You need a little time to get a true feel for the art. Also, you might find an interesting book about Tai Chi — and congratulations! You already have done that part. (My marketing guy told me to say that.)

Fair warning, though: For some folks, Tai Chi can become a way of life. Its mysteries can become a source of fascination. This will develop over time.

Qi Gong

Many people who have heard of Tai Chi may have also heard of Qi Gong. And while there are similarities between them, they are different arts. Qi Gong is the practice of cultivating Qi energy. It is not a martial art. Instead, Qi Gong comprises collections of exercises designed to cultivate the circulation of Qi energy throughout the body. It also promotes health by developing awareness of breath, stretching the fascia, and encouraging relaxation. In many respects, however, Qi Gong is very similar to Tai Chi.

There are many different collections or sets of Qi Gong exercises. Different ones focus on a variety of intentions and outcomes. Some sets are meant to develop balance, flexibility, and strength in the ligaments and tendons. Other sets focus on primarily on cultivating Qi energy flow throughout the body. Still others are used as meditative tools to develop the mind. Some forms of Qi Gong gently compress and release internal organs — and sometimes even the bones. Doing so helps the body to release sedimentary and stagnant liquids and waste.[4] In essence, Qi Gong can have a very similar effect as a good morning stretch. It can relieve tightness and stiffness from inactivity, restore blood and lymphatic fluid flow, and facilitate nerve impulse energy. It also, of course, promotes the circulation of Qi energy.

There are many varieties and collections of individual moves. With Qi Gong, the only things you have to memorize are the moves you wish to practice. You can go to a Qi Gong class taught by a good teacher and follow along fairly easily. On the other hand, Qi Gong won't teach you self-defense, footwork, or moving from one posture to the next. Qi Gong has nothing to offer about interacting with other people. Martial arts applications, if any, offered by Qi Gong are deeply buried and very difficult to find.

With Qi Gong, it is possible to mix and match the exercises you practice as you like. However, for the greatest effect and for purposes of practice and ritual, it is wise to complete all of the exercises in a particular set instead of mixing and matching. This is because each move in a given set is designed to complement all the others and each has a specific purpose that affects the entire body. Some moves in a given set have elements that counter other moves. In other words, a deep forward bend of one kind or another is more effective when

4   Yang, Jwing Ming, The Root of Chinese Qigong: Secrets for Health, Longevity, and Enlightenment, 1997.

it is countered by gently arching the back. Each move complements the whole set.

In the next chapter, we will meet a man called Da Mo. He was an East Indian holy man who lived in the sixth century CE. He traveled to China and ended up at the Shaolin Temple there. He created two Qi Gong sets and a Kung Fu practice. His first Qi Gong set, called Yi Jin Jing, is still widely practiced today. And while there are some variations, it most commonly includes twelve different exercises. Each move focuses on a different motion and a different part of the body. If you are mindful, by the time you finish the entire set, there isn't a part of the body that hasn't received attention. The same can be said for other Qi Gong sets such as Eight Pieces of Brocade or Shibashi, an 18-move set.

Think of Qi Gong like this. When we wake up in the morning or stand up after sitting for a long time and stretch, our body know exactly what kind of stretch it needs. It feels good. Qi Gong tries, in part, to mimic that. With respect to the body, Qi Gong will help you develop flexibility, not only in the sense of expanding range of motion but also in promoting tissue health and elasticity. This includes all of the obvious tissues, such as muscle fibers and so on. It also includes all of the connective tissues, tendons, ligaments; the fascia. Our muscles and our fascia have a particular quality of elasticity depending on how much we move. Fascia fibers stretch and contract. This gives us flexibility. As we get older, the fascia gradually become stiff and brittle. Furthermore, as we age, muscle fibers take on a particular protein, a type of collagen that is also stiff and inelastic. This not only restricts range of motion, but it gives the impression that the body is constricting, curling up, and becoming stiff. Imagine a leaf in the fall, falling from its tree. It becomes brittle and curls up in a different direction than when it was green and vibrant. The constriction of these tissues tugs on the muscles and organs they connect, and that has a restricting effect on blood and energy flow, nerve impulse conduction, and organ functioning.

Qi Gong is quite different than what we think of as "stretching" in the West. The common Western view uses stretching as a means for warming up the muscles in preparation for the "real workout" or for extending our range of motion. We try really hard to touch our toes, for example. Instead, Qi Gong can easily be the "real workout." Though it is a different. Like Tai Chi, Qi Gong wants to integrate your body, mind, and energy. With Qi Gong, extend gently and slowly and feel what is happening inside. Feel what the stretch is doing and trying to tell you. Don't forget to breathe into the stretch. With Qi Gong, most of the time, we want to inhale as we expand. We want to create space in the lungs for more air. With the breath, we want to move energy. Qi Gong also seeks to open various joints and energetic pathways. By doing so, we can facilitate the movement of energy and blood and other fluids throughout the body.

Later on, we will talk about the Fabric Model of the body, which is an idea given to me by Neil B. Anderson, who is a local practitioner of internal martial arts. For now, it is enough to say that all of the various parts of the body, organs, muscles, vessels, bones, etc. are sheathed in fibers called fascia and woven into a fabric. Occasionally, some of the threads or parts of the fabric become twisted, tangled, pinched, or stuck together. Qi Gong might help to put everything back in its proper place. We want the fabric of the body to be organized so that it can promote things like circulation, nervous energy conduction, digestion, lymphatic fluid circulation, and of course, Qi.

Think of the spine, for example. A strong and healthy spine promotes a strong and healthy body. The spine is the information superhighway for the nervous system and all its parts. The spine does not represent an energy meridian, per se. However, there are several meridians that are associated with it. The spine also passes through several energy centers which are associated with meridians and are analogous to the chakra energy centers associated with yoga. Flexibility in the spine and hips means that we can move more efficiently without straining the muscles, fascia, and nerves that extend into the arms and legs. Qi Gong explores the movement and flexibility of the spine along its various rotation vectors.

Comparing Tai Chi and Qi Gong

Many people believe that Qi Gong is part of the Tai Chi universe. I suspect this is because they have heard of or seen Tai Chi. They are vaguely acquainted with it. Also, maybe their Tai Chi teacher includes Qi Gong in class, too. My teacher does. I do, too. Others argue that Tai Chi is instead a subset of Qi Gong.[5] While this is an interesting idea to explore, I believe that Tai Chi and Qi Gong are two separate, interrelated arts. Both can benefit in one or more of the five categories mentioned above: body, breath, Qi cultivation, engaging the mind and cognitive functioning, and developing and enhancing spiritual awareness. Both arts seem to approach each of these categories in different ways.

While both of these arts can enhance your spiritual awareness, neither Tai Chi nor Qi Gong represent any sort of religion. They will not interfere with any sacred beliefs, rituals, or practice you may cherish in any way.

The Book of Changes

Consider the I Ching for a moment.[6] The I Ching has long been considered to be a book of divination — or an oracle. But that has a different meaning than one might expect. We typically think of such things as tools for predicting the future, as if a fortune teller is predicting the intersection of your path and some other external event: "You will meet a tall, dark, handsome stranger." Or "Beware the Ides of March!" That is not the I Ching. There is no prediction, no prognostication or prophesy. Instead, it will shed light on a question you ask of it. It won't chart your path, but it will offer insight on how to proceed. If you let it, it will ask you to look at your question in somewhat of a different light. It's not predictive, it's transformative. It

---

5   Yang, Jwing Ming, Taijiquan, Classical Yang Style: The Complete Form and Qigong, 1999.

6   Wilhelm, The I-Ching, or Book of Changes, 1997.

isn't the sort of thing that lets you take a passive point of view either. It won't tell you what's going to happen to you. Instead, it asks you to think deeply about your question, and it gives you an answer that requires you to look in the mirror. It has a well-deserved reputation for showing you what's already in your head and in your heart. It asks you to consider the sorts of wisdom that you might already possess deep inside but that are simply too clouded by ego or by self for you to see clearly.

The I Ching invites you to ask it a question (one at a time). Then, by casting stalks of yarrow or tossing coins, which are the traditional methods (Although phone apps are also now available), you randomly select one of 64 hexagrams. Each hexagram offers information, additional commentaries, and features. The answers are metaphorical and archetypal. They require you to draw connections between what is offered and what you seek to understand. It's called The Book of Changes because it is transformative. It can guide the way you think about your question. It might ask you to reconsider your perspective. It confronts you with a reflection of yourself. Of course, there is far more that could be said about the I Ching. Endless numbers of books of explanation and commentary have already been written about it. The only real question to be discussed here is this: What does this have to do with Tai Chi?

Very simply stated, the I Ching suggests a cosmology that consists of heaven, earth, and human beings in between. Heaven is represented by Yin. Earth is represented by Yang. Humans embodies the link and the balance between opposing energies. They have both an earthly or base nature comprised of appetites, basic needs, instincts, bodily drives, and also a higher, more spiritual energy. These include the drives of the soul, connection to other human beings, compassion, the meaning of life, and the contemplation of his place in the universe. One energy grounds him in the every day and the other lifts the spirit. The Earthly body fears impermanence — that is death as the end of its journey. The spirit or soul does not. It knows it is eternal. But we don't always listen to it. The I Ching at its most fundamental level, confronts us with these and other questions and asks that we contemplate them deeply.

The Book of Changes, the I-Ching, says that everything began with "the Great Ultimate" or the "Taiji". Maybe, generally speaking, this means God? The Void? The Cosmic Force? From there, the book says, everything separated into two opposing but intertwined and related forces: Yin and Yang. The energy that powers all of this is referred to as Qi, or Chi.

Tai Chi Chuan borrows its name from this idea of the Great Ultimate" in the I Ching Tai Chi Chuan is commonly translated as "Great Ultimate Fist." From a purely marketing perspective, that would be quite the brand identification. "Are you interested in martial arts? Study the Great Ultimate Fist! Sign up today!" Maybe every would-be warrior would want to study the Taiji. Maybe they should. However, that would be a cosmic-sized irony because Tai Chi is an internal art and not commonly expected to be an effective or efficient martial art.[7] That is a mistake. Forgetting the martial arts nature of Tai Chi would be like finding a buried treasure chest, leaving the treasure behind, and only taking the chest.

Consider this: if instead, we think of Tai Chi in those terms, what would that be like? Suddenly, "Great Ultimate" does not modify "fist." It's the other way around. The fist belongs to the Great Ultimate. Thinking about it this way, maybe the fist becomes humanity's way of interacting with the Great Ultimate or the Art of the Cosmos. It begins to represent a search, a quest for humanity's great ultimate connection to the universe.

And so, what if we meant the phrase as a way to explore humanity's relationship to the Great Ultimate? To celebrate our consciousness with respect to the cosmos? What if we thought of Tai Chi as a platform from which to explore human potential? Or cognitive functioning? Or the expansion of consciousness? Or spiritual awareness?

---

7   If you wish to learn how to fight, Krav Maga, the combat system of the Israel Defense Force, or Kenpo are both efficient and very effective.

Perhaps the I Ching works by presenting us with a mirror. It asks us to sit with ourself and reflect on the relationship between the archetypal, primal impulses of ourself and the cosmos. What is our place in the universe? Tai Chi offers us a similar mirror and asks us to reflect on ourself, our relationship to our fellow human beings, and to the Cosmos. Who am I, and who are you?

Yin and Yang

In The Book of Changes, the I Ching, we find this general cosmology: The "Grand Ultimate," the Taiji, was born in the void, or Wuji. Taiji split into two opposing energy constructs: Yin and Yang. These are complementary and dynamic opposing elements. The yin-yang symbol is a graphic description of the Dao — the Way, which is the central governing force of the indigenous Chinese spiritual philosophy called Daoism or Taoism. In addition to the I Ching, The yin-yang symbol is also associated with the Dao Te Ching, written by Chinese philosopher Lao Tzu; and other philosophical works. The Yin Yang symbol is so common, it's almost cliched. It certainly has something to tell us about the art. It has for centuries been associated with Tai Chi. In fact, it is often referred to as the Tai Chi symbol.

The symbol itself demonstrates more than just the interplay of opposing forces (light and dark, for example). Supposing that the Yin Yang symbol, the Taiji, means that things are either black or white misses the point entirely. That perspective is mechanistic, and it unnecessarily reduces the whole into its component halves. Even trying to add gray areas between the black and white only reinforces the error in interpretation. The Yin Yang represents a different perspective entirely. It is a two-dimensional representation of forces in continuous dynamic relationship with each other.

Sifu describes the Yin Yang symbol as two fish endlessly circling each other. Both of them are connected, and both mirror each other. As they move, one fades into the other. Within each can be found an element of the other — an eye, a dot of the other color. The point that he is trying to make is that the relationship between the two is not static. It's dynamic. These two forces always move. As one ebbs, the other flows. Both exist only in relationship to each other. And so the Yin Yang becomes a stylistic representation of the universe.

Yin Yang also refers to the interrelationship of energy and form. Energy, which is lighter, rises, and form, which is heavier, falls. At the same time, both are related. The yin-yang symbol is commonly meant to depict the relationship between any two opposing things or ideas. Indeed, in Western thinking, we talk quite a bit about dualities and dialectics. Many concepts have their polar opposites and engage in a sort of push-pull relationship with each other. Examples of these include light and dark, god and devil, god and human, masculine and feminine, and so on. The Chinese ideogram for yang also means "the sunny side" of the hill or river bank. The ideogram for yin means "the shady side."[8]

There is a relationship between the archetypal energies of masculine and feminine. These energies are a different conversation from talking about gender identification and sexual orientation. These energies are present to varying degrees in every person. Without both yin and yang, there would be no desire for physical or emotional intimacy. However, the yin-yang symbol also is meant to remind us that within every duality, the two opposites comprise a single, unified whole. There is no real distinction between energy and form—they are variations of the same essence. Matter is energy congealed. Masculine and feminine come together to create something new: the continuation of life and meaning. It may not be a common idea in Western thought, but with respect to the duality between god and devil, for example, the two go together. We cannot have a devil without the Author of Everything. Without understanding the forces that bedevil our lives, we would have far less interest in the wisdom of redemption, absolution, mercy, and morality. Putting these opposites together, we understand more

---

8   Veith, The Yellow Emperor's Classic of Internal Medicine, 2002.

about humanity and how to create resilience and post-traumatic growth. With respect to light and dark, you can not see one without the other.

Likewise, within Tai Chi, there is both the knowledge to hurt and the knowledge to heal. Without understanding the process of pain and damage, we cannot understand the process of healing. If we understand healing, then we become much more precise and empathetic about how much harm we cause to others. We learn to moderate and control the damage we inflict so that it meets the needs of defense for ourselves and those we care about and no more.

The Yin Yang is also suggestive of paradox and irony: You can not define an idea without consideration of its opposite. In all things, there is advantage and disadvantage. Of course, strength may overcome softness, but softness may also overcome strength. In all things, there is entropy and decay. There is also growth and adaptation. Every discipline, including martial arts, and Tai Chi in particular, is dependent on the traditions that define it. At the same time, every one also depends on creativity, innovation, and artistic expression (breaking the rules) in order to grow and develop. These are all opposite forces that interact with each other and define each other in sharp contrast.

There is an old Tai Chi maxim: "Only four ounces of effort are needed to deflect a thousand pounds of force." That is, it only takes four ounces if they are applied correctly. Softness can overcome the strong. Patience can overcome aggression. Calm can overcome rage. Stillness is the mother of movement. Ironic, yes. Two sides of the same coin. This is Tai Chi.

With respect to Tai Chi, here are some other paradoxes:

- Letting go of attachment to outcomes is the key to overcoming adversity.

- Be willing to lose in order to win.

- Be willing to receive your opponent's strike in order to dissolve it.

- Listen to your opponent in order to make your point or connect your strike.

- Move quietly in order to make the most impact.

- Practice slowly, intentionally, and be relaxed, and the speed will be free.

- You don't have to be the fastest. You just have to get there first.

- In order to master Tai Chi, you must practice your forms every day, but the form is not Tai Chi.

- Be willing to teach in order to learn.

- Know your opponent, but do not let him know you.

- If it ever feels like you are fighting a ghost, prepare to die. Or learn to fight like a ghost and live.

- Tai Chi is a journey of no destination.

- Tai Chi is the understanding of paradox.

These are all part of a game of riddles that my teacher taught me about Tai Chi. Some, we will look at more in later pages. Others may be for your own contemplation.

Chapter 2: The History of Tai Chi

I suspect that the origin stories of all martial arts systems are heavily influenced by the historical events that gave birth to them. For example, the Israeli combat system Krav Maga was created as a system of street fighting by Jewish resistance fighters in Europe during the twentieth century. They needed a combat system that was effective and relatively easy to learn. After the founding of the state of Israel, Krav Maga was adopted and adapted for training its military troops. Aikido, on the other hand, has its historical roots on the battlefields of ancient Japan. It was originally designed as a system for samurai who had lost their swords and had to face armed and armored opponents. It was burnished and evolved into the "Art of Peace" in the years following World War II during the American occupation of Japan.

For their part, the Chinese are fond of saying that their martial arts and the internal development of Qi energy find their roots deep in the mists of time, going back thousands of years. Tai Chi Chuan began as a tiny little martial art hidden away in the mountains of China, with an idea that was both profound and revolutionary among the arts. That is softness, quiet movement, and connection with your opponent could overcome harshness, strength, and insistence. The flowering, crystallization, and popularization of the art didn't come about until centuries later, during an era of cultural upheaval in China. With respect to the mists of time, however, one historian, Douglas Wile, points out that in the historical accounts of Tai Chi, in particular, there is little certainty regarding the facts and dates.[9] The variation of details among otherwise credible accounts bears this out.

The historical sketch that I present to you here is by no means intended to be comprehensive. There are far more masters, teachers, innovators, writers, and their stories than can possibly be included here. My selection is representational, subjective, and centered firmly on the transmission of the classical Yang-Style tradition, which is only one of several important and well-known Tai Chi traditions. Many of the names and stories I wish to tell you seem to be, in some respects, standard fare for books about Tai Chi. I have worked to ferret out the details, flesh out the stories, and discuss what how they might add to our understanding of the art and its transmission. Even though my intention is to stick closely to the historical accounts and facts, there is, as I mentioned, considerable variation among sources. What I present here might be considered more "lore" about Tai Chi than anything else.

The Book of Changes

Of course, we begin with a book, and we mentioned The Book of Changes a moment ago. Here is a little of the history. The I Ching, The Book of Changes, is said to be one of the oldest existing books. It has a history that can be traced back some five thousand years or more. It is said to have been invented, or "written," by Fu Xi, who was a progenitor hero of Chinese civilization — you know, one of those semi-mythological or legendary heroes who might be only part human. According to legend, Fu Xi intended The Book of Changes to teach mankind the skills of civilization: hunting, agriculture, cooking, the values of social contract, and so on. However, as time went on, the book evolved into an oracle, a book of divination, magic – or simply, a book of great wisdom.

It didn't exactly begin in any form we might recognize as a book. At the time it is said to have been written, few people could read, and there was little if anything that we might consider as "paper."

---

9   Wile, Tai-Chi Touchstones: Yang Family Secret Transmissions, 1983.

According to the lore, "the book" was at first a collection of line symbols scratched out on bamboo stalks. Some thousands of years later, the I Ching was amended by King Wen and his son, the Duke of Cho. They were the founders of the Cho Dynasty, which began a thousand years before the Common Era. Later still, Confucius, one of China's most influential philosophers, is said to have added commentary to it. He came to the I Ching late in life, when he was old enough to understand it. He is also known for commenting that there was never enough time to study the entire book properly.

The I Ching offers a cosmology that begins with the Taiji, the Great Ultimate, and immediately breaks into two opposite energies: Yin and Yang, which ebb and flow in relationship to each other in an endless circle, always moving. It is the flow of history. So, let us take a look at a few of the historical characters.

Da Mo (483–561 C.E.)

We pick up the more common thread of the origin of Tai Chi in the late fifth century of the Common Era, in India with a Buddhist monk called Da Mo. We know a little bit about him and there is some variation among sources about the dates of his life.[10] We know his family name was Sardili. We know he grew up a prince in a small, regional kingdom in India. He renounced his life of luxury and privilege, as well as his claim to the throne, so that he might follow the path of Buddhist enlightenment. He did not become a Buddha. Instead, he became a Bodhidharma — a man who had renounced the path of personal enlightenment in order to move through the temporal world and bring aid and comfort and perhaps even enlightenment to others.[11] He did apparently possess a keen knowledge of meditation, yoga, and Indian martial arts.

Da Mo was dispatched from India to bring Buddhism to China. He is the second Indian monk recorded as doing so. Ominously,

---

10   Yang, Qigong: The Secret of Youth: Da Mo's Muscle/Tendon Changing and Marrow/Brain Washing Techniques, 2000.

11   Liang, Tai Chi Chuan: 24 and 48 postures with martial applications, 1996.

the first apparently went and never returned. Of course, there is no indication that Da Mo ever returned to India, either. So the story goes.

In learning about Da Mo, one gets the impression that he had an active and restless intellect. There is some evidence to suggest that by the time he arrived at the court of the Chinese emperor, he had already developed his own ideas about the path of Buddhist enlightenment and he may have possessed the stubbornness of an educated missionary.

Da Mo arrived in China about 520 CE. This was a time of flowering and growth of Buddhism in China. At the time, the number of Buddhist monasteries in China grew from about 6,500 or more than 30,000 during the 60 or so years from the late fifth century to the mid-sixth century CE. Da Mo arrived just in the middle of it.[12]

Da Mo presented himself to the court of Emperor Wu of the Liang Dynasty. That meeting between monk and emperor is described nearly the same way in nearly every historical account of Tai Chi that I've seen. They spent some time together, and while there was a meeting of the men, there was no meeting of the minds. Perhaps the Chinese emperor grew tired of the religious prattlings of a foreign monk. One might imagine that men of emperor status are more fond of pomp and ceremony that centers around the royal court and have little stomach for the proselytizing of foreign missionaries. Or perhaps Da Mo lost patience with the likely limited attention span of the politically minded emperor. We just don't know.

However, in what might have been a happy circumstance of history, following his setback at court, Da Mo retired to the Shaolin Temple in Henan Province.[13] There, he found a mystery to which he

---

12 Diepersloot, The Tao Of Yiquan: The Method of Awareness in the Martial Arts, 1999.

13 Yang, Jwing Ming, Qigong: The Secret of Youth: Da Mo's Muscle/Tendon Changing and Marrow/Brain Washing Techniques, Taijiquan, Classical Yang Style: The Complete Form and Qigong, 2000.

could apply his intellect. He found that the monks subscribed to a particular philosophy that centered around cultivating their spiritual minds through prayer and meditation, but they were disdainful and dismissive of the physical body. In the absence of a healthy mind-body connection, they were weak and sickly. They didn't have the strength or stamina to conduct their daily prayers and meditations without falling asleep. Their physical limitations affected their ability to cultivate their spiritual minds.

According to the story, Da Mo either retired to a cave or sat before a wall to meditate on the problem. After some years, some sources say nine[14], he emerged from his cave bearing three revolutionary training methods. The first was a series of hand gestures which became "Eighteen Buddha Boxing Method" or "Eighteen Ways of the Warrior Monks"[15] This became the progenitor of Shaolin Gong Fu.

The other two training methods that he introduced were very specialized forms of Qi Gong. Qi Gong is the study of energy circulation exercises in the body. Da Mo's first Qi Gong manuscript focused on strengthening the tendons and ligaments, something he saw as promoting strength, stamina, and vitality. The second focused on developing longevity. According to legend, if it was practiced properly, this second form would lead to enlightenment but only in concert with the foundation of the first one. The first, called Yi Jin Jing, is "The Classic on Muscle and Ligament Strengthening." The second is called Xi Sui Jing, "The Classic on Bone Marrow Washing."[16] Some sources suggest that Da Mo was the first to match meditation, breathing, and Qi energy cultivation techniques with external fighting techniques. We still have arguably accurate versions of Da Mo's works on Qi Gong, and many people continue to study them today. With Da Mo's training, the monks at the Shaolin Temple

---

14   Yang, Jwing Ming, Taijiquan, Classical Yang Style: The Complete Form and Qigong, 1999.

15   Dieppersloot, 1999.

16   Yang, Jwing-Ming, 1999.

refocused their efforts on cultivating the mind and the body and the monks quickly became reinvigorated. So the story goes.

Eventually, Da Mo's philosophies about Ch'an Buddhism and the importance of the mind- body connection became a foundational philosophy in Chinese martial arts. These ideas spread across China and eventually they spread across the seas to Japan where they became known as Zen Buddhism and were integrated as a core philosophy of the traditional Japanese martial arts as well.[17]

Cheng San Feng (1274 –?)

We move here from the Buddhists to the early Daoists, and that brings us to perhaps one of the more famous, more colorful figures in Tai Chi lore. Cheng San Feng was something of a mysterious, mystical figure: a Daoist sage, a monk, an alchemist, something of a wild man, something of a hermit, and possibly an immortal. All this he became—at least in the pages of Chinese history.

Cheng San Feng was born at midnight on April 9, 1247.[18] He is commonly described as having the back of a turtle and the neck of a crane. He might have been seven feet tall. He had large round eyes, and many believed that meant he was born wise. It is also said that at times, he could go months without eating and then devour monstrous portions of food in a single sitting. He presented a robust figure, perhaps even portly. He had long, unkempt hair and a beard hat was often stained with the juice of wild berries.[19] It might have been said about him: "That wizard is just a crazy old man." Maybe. He was also nicknamed "Sloppy Cheng" because he did not pay a lot of attention to personal hygiene. Like many figures half obscured by time, the shadow of the legend might be taller than the man himself.

---

17 Yang, Jwing-Ming, 2000.

18 Jou, The Tao of Tai-Chi Chuan: Way to Rejuvenation, 1991. Given the variation of details surrounding this mysterious figure or figures, this appears a rather bold statement. However, Jou points out that the anniversary of Cheng San Feng's birth is still celebrated. In the US as World Tai Chi Day.

19 Yang Jwing Ming, 1999.

Still, when it comes to the lore of Tai Chi, the name of Cheng San Feng is well remembered.

Cheng San Feng had been a monk at the Shaolin Temple for 10 years.[20] There, he had mastered hard, external fighting styles. One day he left—for who knows what reason. It might be that Cheng San Feng was critical of the kind of training the monks there had been receiving. Perhaps he thought something was missing. Maybe he figured there was something more to learn. It might be suggested that by then, the physical discipline presented by Da Mo had grown out of fashion. Perhaps Chang San Feng grew restless and wished to improve what they were already learning. Perhaps he longed to revise or contribute the monks' understanding of the fighting arts.

Whatever the reason, Cheng San Feng left the Shaolin Temple for Wudang Mountain. Various stories suggest that he wandered, that he lived in huts made of grass. Other stories say he found caves in which to meditate. After some years, the answer to his search came to him. It was his custom to rise with the rising sun. On one particular morning, he happened to watch a snake emerge from its hole. A bird was intent upon the snake as well. Some stories say it was a crane. Others suggest it was a magpie. In either case, the bird was looking for breakfast, and it had its eye on the snake. The bird swooped down to attack, and a furious battle ensued. Cheng San Feng watched intently. The bird jabbed with its sharp beak, and the snake circled and coiled to escape the beaky jabs. The snake was successful in fending off the crane. The episode had a profound effect on the thinking of our hermit. It inspired him to rethink the fighting arts of Shaolin. The battle he watched became the inspiration for Tai Chi Chuan.[21]

In another story, Cheng San Feng somehow attracted the attention of the Song dynasty Emperor Hui Tsung and he had been

---

20 Jou, 1991.

21 Jou, 1991. This is the only account of that story that I have ever seen which declares a victory to one side or the other.

summoned to the imperial court. On his way there, he found that the road had been blocked by bandits. Unable to proceed, he retired to make camp. That night, he dreamt that the Daoist deity Yuan-Ti had taught him martial arts. The next day, Cheng San Feng fought and defeated more than a hundred bandits. He continued on his way to the palace.

In yet another story, Cheng San Feng spent a great deal of time wandering throughout the Wudang mountains meditating and searching for wisdom. According to some accounts, he was very much attuned to the natural world around him. Animals would warn him of danger, and he was known for battling boa constrictors and tigers with his bare hands. It has been said that among his greatest disciples was an ape that Cheng San Feng had trained in the postures of Tai Ch Chuan.[22]

The story suggests that Cheng San Feng didn't learn the secrets of becoming a Daoist immortal until his early 70s; that he didn't actually become immortal until he was nearly 80. He was much older than that when the Ming dynasty began in 1368.[23] Indeed, by then he would already have been 120.

Cheng San Feng was always wary of attracting the attention of the imperial court, and yet still, somehow, he did. So he spent years playing hide and seek with court officials who were sent to find him and press him into service. He even pretended to be mad and wore the nickname "Sloppy Cheng" in hopes the imperials would hear about his reputation and become disgusted and dissuaded from continuing their search.

According to the lore, Cheng San Feng lived variously more than two hundred years or more than five hundred years. Some scholars wrote that he was "immortal." Others attribute his apparent longevity to fact that there were two different Cheng San Fengs who lived centuries apart but who were thought to be the same man. The

---

22   Jou, 1991.

23   Jou, 1991.

first was the famous Daoist sage of the Song Dynasty. He was Cheng "of Three Mountain Peaks." Many of the famous stories are about him. The second was Cheng "of Three Abundances" and he likely lived later, during the Ming Dynasty.[24] The first Cheng San Feng eventually settled in the Pao Gi mountains in Central China which are said to have three peaks or "San Feng."[25]

Yet another story attributes Cheng San Feng's longevity to covert political intrigues. In a story reminiscent of Shakespeare's Hamlet, during the Ming Dynasty, there was a man called Jian Wen who was crown prince. Within a short span of years, both his grandfather, who had long been emperor, and his father, who held the throne only briefly, died. As one might imagine, this opened the way to the throne for the prince. Instead, Jian Wen's uncle, Yong Le, usurped the throne, and Jian Wen was forced to flee the capital in fear of his life.

Fearing that his nephew would one day gather power and return to wrest away the throne, Yong Le sent assassins to scour the empire in search of him, but he needed a cover story to disguise his nefarious intent. So Yong Le claimed he was sending out search parties in search of a famous Daoist immortal called Cheng San Feng. By then, of course, Cheng San Feng had been a folk hero for many years, but no one had actually seen him (possibly because he had died many many years before). Yong Le's assassins searched the empire for more than 20 years. They never found Jian Wen, and they never found Cheng San Feng. To further conceal his true intent, Yong Le had a temple built in the Wudang mountains in honor of this "immortal sage." It has been suggested that stories and rumors about this search for Cheng San Feng made it appear as though the man had lived for centuries. In essence, according to those stories, Cheng San Feng may have owed his considerable longevity to little more than political conspiracies.

---

24 Huang, Complete Tai-Chi: The Definitive Guide to Physical and Emotional Self-Development, 1997.

25 Jou, 1991.

Still, the most popular stories about Cheng San Feng's exploits in martial arts and his longevity suggest that despite the incredible length of time between the two Cheng San Fengs, that both were in fact the same man.

Wile notes, "If Cheng San Feng did not exist as the father of Tai Chi Ch'uan, it would be necessary to invent him. Most of the martial arts in China boast mythopoetic beginnings; it is simply a convention. Starry-eyed students would feel cheated by pedestrian accounts of sweaty men punching each other around the back yard."[26]

Still, it was Immortal Cheng San Feng who matched Qi energy cultivation with breathing techniques and philosophies from the Daoist Book of Changes, the I Ching, to the teachings at the Shaolin Temple.[27] Perhaps, based on the story of the snake and the crane, he became inspired to add the softness, quiet movements. strikes, and circles that we attribute to contemporary Tai Chi. Maybe that is true.

Chen Wang Ting (1597–1664)

Our next character is alive during the dying days of the Ming dynasty some years following Cheng San Feng's exit from our stage. Chen Wang Ting[28] is said to have learned his fighting style directly from one of the disciples of Cheng San Feng.[29] He is remembered as the patriarch of the ninth generation of the Chen family. Some accounts claim that today's Chen family still possesses a saber that Chen Wang Ting once carried in battle.[30] He was a military man; a

---

26 Wile, Tai-Chi Touchstones: Yang Family Secret Transmissions, 1983. Translator's Note.

27 Jou, 1991.

28 In Asian cultures, including Japan and China, it is common to place a person's family name first, followed by their given or familiar name. Chen Wang Ting is a member of the Chen family. His family likely called him simply Ting.

29 Jou, 1991.

30 Huang, 1993.

garrison commander in Wen County during late Ming Dynasty.[31] He was also reputed to escort trade caravans an protect them against bandits. He is credited with winning a battle in Shantung Province against more than a thousand invaders. Presumably, he had some help.

In any case, when the Ming Dynasty fell in 1644 CE, Chen Wang Ting retired to the family estate in Chen Village in Henan Province to study literature and martial arts. He became the founder of Chen's Fist, Hand, Saber, and Spear Martial Arts. It is said that Chen Wang Ting was, in fact, the first to combine matched-breathing techniques with previous ideas about physical postures in Chinese martial arts. He is credited with updating prior ideas about external techniques of hands, feet, and body with the internal breathing system and Qi circulation developed by the Daoist monks. Chen is likewise credited with introducing the cultivation of Chi internal energy and Jin (Jing), the physical expression of Qi. In other words, Chen is credited with the entire internal framework of Tai Chi.[32]

Chen Wang Ting passed his martial arts legacy down through generations of Chen family. According to the common thread of Tai Chi lore, the next off shoot would take place during the fourteenth generation of the Chen family when a man called Yang Lu Chan appeared. Before we get to that, though, we should note that even today, Chen Style Tai Chi is as robust and well known as ever. It remains one of the most important branches of Tai Chi and is still commonly practiced. However, our historical account takes a different turn.

Yang Lu Chan (1799–1872)

The Yang family enters the story of Tai Chi Chuan with Yang Lu Chan. He was born into a farming family in Hubei Province. He became a servant in the house of Chen Ch'ang-Hsing, a direct

---

31   Huang, 1993.

32   Huang, 1993.

descendant of Chen Wang Ting. Yang Lu Chan wanted to study martial arts and found his way into the Chen family to steal their treasures. Specifically, he wanted to learn their secret fighting techniques. However, they did not generally share their secrets with outsiders. One night, after serving in the Chen household for some years, Yang Lu Chan heard the sounds of men training in martial arts. He discovered a way to spy on these secret training classes by peeking through a crack in a wall, or perhaps through a window. It became his daily routine to spy on the secret class and retire to his room to practice what he had seen. And so his skills grew in secret.

Later, in a scene that must have inspired many future Kung Fu Theater melodramas, a man appeared at the Chen family home and challenged the Chen master, Chen Ch'ang-Hsing, to a "friendly" fight. This was a common practice across China as a way to test the validity and strength of the family system of martial arts. The challenge could not be ignored. Chen's most skilled disciple was sent to answer the challenge and was soundly thrashed. The man repeated his challenge to Chen Ch'ang-Hsing, and again, it could not be ignored. However, if Chen lost, it would be a tremendous blow to the credibility of the Chen family. It would mean a loss of face. This is where we get the sense of rising drama. Who would step up to protect the master and the family tradition?

Of course, Yang Lu Chan stepped up to answer the challenge: "I am a simple servant with little understanding of the art. Would you, sir, allow me to learn a little from you in friendly competition?" The man accepted Yang Lu Chan's challenge, and the two fought. Yang Lu Chan won the fight handily using the Chen family techniques that he had learned in secret.

But there was a problem. During that time in China, the theft by an outsider of a family's secret fighting techniques was punishable by death. These fighting techniques were closely guarded secrets. Knowing this, Yang Lu Chan presented himself to Master Chen Ch'ang-Hsing for judgement and offered him tea. He knew the gravity of the situation. It was very likely he would be put to death.

However, the Chen master accepted the tea and gave this reply: "Yang Lu Chan has saved our family's honor. He is not an outsider. He is my servant, and by drinking this tea he has offered, I have accepted him as my disciple." And so, Yang Lu Chan was saved and became a trusted disciple.

Yang Lu Chan continued for some years to study with the Chen Family. Later, he returned to his home where he taught others what he had learned. He fought many challenges and never lost. He became known as "Unbeatable Yang". There are many stories describing how Yang Lu Chan went to great lengths, took great risks, and exercised great skill to save his opponents from undue injury; from falling off a battlement, for example. The stories vary widely, and Yang Lu Chan left no personal writings behind to corroborate these legends.[33] However, as far as reputations go, many years later, when he was teaching his own sons the art, he became known as a very demanding and difficult teacher.[34]

But before we get in to that, there is one other piece of lore to look at. Yang Lu Chan caught the attention of the Qing dynasty emperor and received an invitation to share his art with the imperial court and guard. Of course such an invitation was not something one could easily decline. By all accounts, Yang Lu Chan was less than enamored by the situation. Some say he found the imperial court less than equal to the discipline and athleticism required by the art. Others suggest that his reluctance was due to political or tribal differences with the Qing dynasty. The Qings were Manchus, after all, a tribe from the north. They were considered to be foreigners and invaders.

According to some stories, members of the imperial family did not possess the athletic ability, stamina, or motivation to learn the same curriculum that Yang Lu Chan taught to the imperial guards. Yang Lu Chan was not too fond of the imperial family, and so he withheld some of the finer details and techniques of Tai Chi. The

---

33 Wile, 1996

34 Liang, Tai Chi Chuan: 24 and 48 postures with martial applications, 1996.

imperial family was taught a version of Tai Chi intended to promote health and wellness. Of course, the imperial guard wanted to learn the art in order to win battles.

In any case, at the imperial court, Yang Lu Chan presented a version of Tai Chi Chuan that was stripped of its more difficult moves—leaps and kicks and so on. This version focused on developing health and well-being instead of martial prowess, and it was this version of Tai Chi Chuan that became the classical, or large-frame, Yang Style of Tai Chi that is very popular today. The secrets that Yang Lu Chan withheld became the Secret or Michuan Yang Style. It is also called "small frame." For several generations, these teachings became reserved for family and trusted disciples. Although, today, it can still be found.

Certainly if the Qing imperials learned that Yang Lu Chan had withheld secrets from them, there would have been trouble. At the same time, there was a trove of information that needed to be preserved. It must have presented quite the conundrum, and there was quite a lot at stake.

Perhaps it is easy to imagine why Yang Lu Chan could have been such a difficult teacher. One gets the impression that he was an extremely skilled martial artist and burdened with a great responsibility. He clearly had much to contribute to the art. When it came to passing along his prodigious understanding to his sons, it had to be done precisely and quietly. It wouldn't do to have the wrong people learn that Yang Lu Chan had withheld secrets. Let's add one more thought to the mix: sometimes, the sons of gifted men find their father to be less than patient with them when it comes to passing along the family legacy. There is some evidence to suggest that this may have been the case here. Among his three sons, one died as an infant. The other two carried on the legacy Yang Lu Chan began. This brings us to the next notable man in our story: Yang Lu Chan's grandson, Yang Chen Fu.

Yang Chen Fu (1883–1936)

Yang Lu Chan never knew his grandson, Yang Chen Fu. He died 11 years before the younger man was born.[35] Yang Chen Fu was greatly influenced by the cultural upheaval taking place during the transition from the late nineteenth century through the opening years of the twentieth century. His greatest impact was made during the 1920s and 30s.[36] He is credited with transforming an indigenous, clan-transmitted system of self-defense and well-being into a national cultural treasure.

During his relatively short life, Yang Chen Fu witnessed the first Sino-Japanese war in 1894. He also saw the birth of the short-lived Chinese Republic and the gathering storm clouds between them and the Chinese Communists.

It appears as though his interest in Tai Chi was to help his countrymen reclaim their strength, vigor, and dignity.[37] Yang Chen Fu did not begin his studies of Tai Chi until his twenties, which was considerably late for the times, especially considering his family legacy. He began to study in earnest when "he realized Tai Chi could not only improve his own health, but also cultivate the whole nation's physical condition and awaken the spirit of the entire country."[38]

Like his famous grandfather, Yang Chen Fu became a sought-after teacher. Unlike his grandfather, Yang Chen Fu did not seem to have the same interest in testing his prowess against challengers. Perhaps he was an idealistic man. It was said that he had a kind nature and was a more patient teacher than his grandfather. Indeed,

---

35 Yang, Chengfu. The Essence and Applications of Taijiquan, 2005. There is a passage in Yang Chen Fu's 1934 book that describes watching his grandfather Yang Lu Chan leading other extended family members in a Tai Chi Chuan practice. However, it is commonly accepted that Chen Fu was born about eleven years after Lu Chan died.

36 Yang Chengfu, 2005. Also, Wile, 1983.

37 Wile, 1996.

38 Jou, 1991, p. 46

he is considered to be one of the greatest Tai Chi teachers ever.[39] As a younger man, he was diligent in his daily practice. Later on, other things took priority. He grew old and fat before his time and less flexible in executing his technique. He died in his fifties.[40]

At least three generations of Yang Family taught Tai Chi in the Qing imperial court. Yang Chen Fu taught the Yang Large Frame style. He is credited with creating the Yang Style 108 posture form. Yang Chen Fu takes the story of Tai Chi into the twentieth century. Yang Chen Fu's aim was to develop a system of Tai Chi suitable for improving the well-being, strength, vigor, and dignity of a nation suffering one existential crisis after another. In 1934, Yang Chen Fu published a revised edition of his 1931 book.[41] Yang Chen Fu's revision, The Essence and Applications of Tai Chi Quan was meant to be a more polished, more accessible distillation of his teaching than the previous version. It was edited by Yang Chen Fu's last disciple, Cheng Man Ching. The book codified and crystalized Yang Chen Fu's thinking about public Tai Chi. This publication became the seed of the Classical Yang Style that remains popular today.

Indeed, the publication of the book marked a turning point in the transmission of Tai Chi. The earlier classic texts were highly codified, privately circulated manuscripts. They were often intentionally obscure and poetic in their language in order to protect the secrets they held. These texts, poems and songs really, did not explain things clearly. They were only intended to jog the memories of masters and advanced students who had already mastered the techniques they described.[42]

Yang Cheng Fu's book, however, was clearly written for the general public. It contains descriptions of each move and explanations of their applications. It is among the earlier — if not the earliest—books about Tai Chi Chuan to make use of photographs demonstrating

---

39   Liang, 1996.

40   Jou, 1991.

41   Yang Chenfu, 2005.

42   Yang Chenfu, 2005.

various postures. The publication of the book became a vehicle that popularized Tai Chi in general and Yang Chen Fu's teaching in particular. It is easy to speculate that the publication of the book contributed greatly to both the flowering of Yang Chen Fu's brand of Tai Chi as well as its spread across China. Wile notes that Tai Chi has become one of the "world's great sciences of self-cultivation"[43] alongside meditation disciplines and yoga, and for that, we have Yang Chen Fu and his book to thank.

Cheng Man Ching (1900–1975)

If it was Yang Chen Fu's destiny to liberate Tai Chi from the clannish, oral transmissions and popularize Tai Chi across Mainland China, it would be Cheng Man Ching who brought the art to Taiwan and the West. Cheng Man Ching studied with Yang Chen Fu for seven years. Later, he ran a school for Tai Chi in New York City from 1965 until his death 10 years later[44].

There is an old story about Cheng Man Ching. As a child, he was quite rambunctious. One day, he was out playing when a wall caved in on him. The details of this accident aren't clear, but we do know it left him unconscious for a time and with lasting cognitive impairments. According to Lowenthal, Cheng Man Ching was awoken from a coma by an itinerant Daoist monk. For years after, he had difficulty concentrating and was expected to suffer permanent brain damage.[45] He restored his brain function by practicing Yi Jin Jing, one of the health and wellness regimens that Da Mo had resented to the Shaolin monks centuries before.[46] Later, Cheng Man Ching suffered from rickets, rheumatism, and tuberculosis. They led him to the study of Tai Chi and saw him returned to health.[47]

---

43 Wile, 1996.

44 Lowenthal, There are no Secrets: Professor Cheng Man-ch'ing and his Tai Chi Chuan, 1991.

45 Lowenthal, 1991.

46 Jou, 1991.

47 Lowenthal, 1991.

There is another especially noteworthy story about Cheng Man Ching. He published a number of books during his life. A couple of years after his teacher Yang Chen Fu died, Cheng Man Ching created his own Simplified 37-Posture Form. In 1949, he published the form in his own book: Master Cheng's New Method of Taichi Ch'uan Self-Cultivation.[48]

Only a few years earlier, Cheng Man Ching had edited the work of his teacher Yang Chen Fu. Yang Chen Fu's book was a compendium of his teachings and thoughts about his brand of Tai Chi. Cheng Man Ching's 37-posture form is quite different from the form created by Yang Chen Fu. As Shakespeare wrote, "The funeral baked meats did coldly furnish forth the wedding table."[49] In other words, although his teacher had just died, Cheng Man Ching was already changing the legacy. To be clear, Cheng Man Ching's 37-Posture Form still had the trappings and taste of a Yang Style form. However it marked a split of traditional Yang Style Tai Chi into two distinct branches.

Sophia Delza (1908–1996)

A quick note about women in Tai Chi. It goes without saying that today there are many extraordinarily talented and knowledgeable women practicing martial arts in general and Tai Chi in particular. With respect to Tai Chi, however, women came later to the stage. There is little mention of women participating in Tai Chi before the mid-twentieth century. You do get occasional legends like the Sword Maiden of Yueh and Mulan. However, gender roles in China were too conservative and calcified. Perhaps clan patriarchs were reluctant to teach family secrets to their daughters because once they got married, any such secrets would become the property of the new husband, and the family would lose control of them. Of course, this began to slowly change during the Chinese Republic Era.

---

48 Cheng, Master Cheng's New Method of Tai Chi Self-Cultivation, 1999.

49 Shakespeare, Hamlet, Prince of Denmark, Act 1, Scene 2.

However, in 1948, an American man called Cook Glassgold left New York City for a diplomatic posting to China. He took along his wife, Sophia Delza. Delza was already well-known in New York as a dancer and choreographer. During the four years that the couple resided in Shanghai, China, Delza became the first American to teach modern dance in theaters and classrooms in China. She also studied Tai Chi with a well-known teacher of the Wu Style[50] called Ma Yueh Liang. Wu Style is a descended from the Yang Style, but the story of its development and flowering is for another time.

When Delza returned to New York in 1951, she began teaching Tai Chi. She opened a school at Carnegie Hall in 1954. That same year, she gave a public dance performance which included a demonstration of Wu Style Tai Chi at the Museum of Modern Art in New York City. It may have been the first public demonstration of Tai Chi in America. Delza also wrote a number of articles and books about Tai Chi. Her 1961 book T'ai Chi Ch'uan: Body and Mind in Harmony is thought to be the first English-language book about Tai Chi. Apparently, Delza was quite the colorful figure during an already colorful time in American history. With respect to our story about Tai Chi in America, she was truly a pioneer.

Tai Chi in the Time of Qing Dynasty (1644 – 1911)

The Qing Dynasty began in 1644 when nomadic Manchu invaders from the north usurped the imperial Ming Dynasty throne. The Qing Dynasty lasted until the dawn of the short-lived Chinese Republic in 1911.[51] Toward the end of the Qing dynasty, though, China fell under siege by from powers from across the seas: Japan, Europe, and the United States. Furthermore, it was a time of radical economic and industrial upheaval — the era of trains, telegraph, and guns. Trains brought people, mechanically produced goods to compete with

---

50   Wu Style is descended from the Yang Style, but the story of its development and flowering is for another time.

51   Yang, 1999.

locally produced counterparts, and foreign ideas about religion and landownership. Telegraphs wired nearly instant information and news from far away places. Guns and military technology flooded in from the West and changed the way battles were fought.

To put it into sharper contrast, Yang Lu Chan was teaching Tai Chi in the age of Darwin, but he also likely watched French and British forces invade the Chinese capital, Peking, and chase away the Manchu Emperor in 1860.[52] This was about the same time as the US Civil War.

His grandson Yang Chen Fu was formulating his philosophy about Tai Chi at the same time that Chinese military units carried European-made rifles on the battlefield. Swords were still carried, but their utility was already greatly diminished.[53] Elsewhere at about the same time, the Wright Brothers completed their first powered flight in 1903, and Albert Einstein had his Miracle Year in 1905 when he unveiled his work on general and special relativity and on Brownian motion.[54] Yang Chen Fu was alive during the first world war and the dawn of mechanized warfare. His most productive years came were during the 1920s and 30s.

This raises a question. Yang Lu Chan was summoned to teach Tai Chi at the Imperial Court and in the military garrisons. Not only that, but the Yang family would continue to teach Tai Chi in the Imperial Court for at least three generations, at least until the fall of the Qing Manchus and the rise of the Chinese Republic. So the question remains: Why? Why was Tai Chi important to the Qing imperials? Wile (1996) suggests that over time, the Qing Manchus were becoming ever more Chinese in their affectations. Perhaps this was due to the gravity well of assimilation from Manchu to Chinese across long generations. Perhaps it was an intentional strategy on the part of the Manchus to appear more like their Chinese subjects as a means to hold onto power. Perhaps it was a little of both.

---

52   Wile, 1996.

53   Wile, 1996.

54   Isaacson, Einstein: His Life and Universe, 2007.

Meanwhile, there is still the mystery of why Tai Chi continued to gain popularity in an age when brawls and battlefields were populated by pistols and rifles. Furthermore, while many Chinese people wholly rejected Western culture and religion, pragmatic Chinese thinkers understood the utility of adopting Western military technology.[55] However, the history books show us that such pragmatic thinking was not enough.

The history books talk quite a bit about the development of Tai Chi as a martial art. There is also robust discussion about Tai Chi as a regimen for cultivating health and well-being. These traditions stretch all the way back to Da Mo, as we have seen. Yang Chen Fu used these traditions to spread Tai Chi.[56]

Maybe there is also a political reason in play. What is talked about considerably less is the notion that Tai Chi served to empower Chinese cultural resilience. Perhaps this is not as speculative an idea as one might think. Tai Chi embodies Chinese cultural notions of calmness and stillness in the face of conflict, using softness to overcome strength, and patience to develop resilience. These represent a Chinese answer to the overwhelming military strength of foreign invaders. We can talk about how these apply to personal combat and conflict, and we will.

We can also apply these same notions to a people who were and perhaps are still looking for meaning in their personal lives in an age of upheaval and hoping for national redemption. Yang Chen Fu argues that Tai Chi is a means of awakening the might and prowess of the Chinese people in their struggles against the Qing Manchus, the Japanese, and the Western powers.[57] If the stories of Tai Chi giants the others are to be believed, and retold, these heroes had to become larger than life: Immortal Cheng San Feng defeated a hundred bandits after dreaming that the god of war taught him

---

55 Wile, 1983.

56 Liang, 1996.

57 Yang Chenfu, 2005. Jou, 1991.

how to fight. Chen Wang Ting was famous in Shantung Province for winning a battle against more than a thousand invaders. Unbeatable Yang never lost a duel while also taking great pains to avoid harming his opponents. Perhaps these stories about Tai Chi heroes are true, but arguing about it misses the point. They have become sources of internal Chinese pride and dignity. These stories were reborn during a particularly tumultuous century that included the decline and overthrow of the Qing dynasty, the rise and fall of the Chinese Republic, and the civil war that saw gave birth to the Chinese Communist Era. There was more. Wars with foreign powers, Japan, Russia, and the West, exploited the weakening Qing Manchus, and converted a proud empire into almost a colonial possession. During this time, the Chinese people were beaten at war, invaded, colonized, and passed around like spoils to the victors. So these stories, even if they are fantasies, these home-grown stories of the indomitable prowess of national heroes offered the promise of hope, dignity, and national redemption.

Return for a moment to our mysterious hero Cheng San Feng. We might imagine that stories about him grew popular during the later Qing Dynasty and Chinese Republic. Cheng San Feng was a legendary Chinese folk hero. His existence and heroic stature can neither be wholly proven nor completely dismissed. Whether or not he is the father of Tai Chi, he is undoubtedly the embodiment of core Tai Chi principles. Whether he acquired his prodigious understanding of Tai Chi by watching nature or through a dream or through years-long meditations on the needs of the Shaolin monks, his story is uniquely Chinese. Even if his story is an allegory or a fairy tale, it can not be overrun, overthrown, or taken away. Chang San Feng remains an avatar of Chinese culture and resilience. From there, Tai Chi becomes a sort of personal internal rebellion against external invaders. And so it becomes somewhat subversive. That is Tai Chi. Perhaps we can use that story to build our own internal resilience in the face of foreign invaders or in the face of challenges in our daily life.

After the Fall of the Qing Dynasty

Yang Chen Fu's teaching, fueled by his popularity and in no small measure by his book, would ride a wave of popularity through the Republic Era and even during the early years of the Chinese Communist Revolution. Wile writes, "Through Yang's [Chen Fu] own genius and the energy and prestige of this students, the 'Yang Style' of T'ai Chi Ch'uan established itself as the dominant internal system in China."[58] Indeed, in 1956, the Chinese National Athletic Association systematized and formalized its version of the 24 Posture form for the expressed purpose of unifying Tai Chi for the entire country and for the more quiet purpose of stripping much of the martial arts applications from the art.[59] It would simply not do to empower the people by teaching them how to fight.

The tides receded in 1966: Tai Chi crashed onto the rocks of the Cultural Revolution and was completely outlawed by the Communist Chinese. Later, in 1976, they seemed to realize they had made a mistake and that Tai Chi, among other things, represented an important part of Chinese cultural heritage. In 1989, they established the Classical Yang Style 48 Posture form (also called the 42 Posture Form). This form incorporated elements from other major styles of Tai Chi: Chen Style, Wu Style, and Sun Style, etc. They wanted to have a common form that could unite the disparate styles in order to promote competition among all Tai Chi practitioners. Later still, they formalized the 16 Posture form and the 8 Posture form. These became the foundation of the Classical Yang Style Tai Chi curriculum for the People's Republic of China.

Also during the fifties, Cheng Man Ching took his 37 Posture form to Taiwan and New York. His teaching came to represent the exported version of the Yang Style. He taught hundreds of students and wrote a number of books until his death in 1975. It should also be noted that despite their differences, Cheng Man Ching and

---

58   Wile, 1983.Translator's note.

59   Liang, 1996.

Yang Chen Fu agreed on the foundational ideas. They both carried forward the foundational philosophies and theories of Tai Chi, the core principles. In addition, they both wished to bring Tai Chi out of the shadows of the family clans and out from behind the gates of the imperial court. Both men believed it was important to bring Tai Chi to the world. Meanwhile, today in China, one Tai Chi historian writes, "For the tens of millions of practitioners in China today, t'ai-chi ch'uan fills the spiritual vacuum left by the collapse of socialist idealism."[60]

There is one more figure I would like to introduce you to. Let's meet my teacher.

---

60   Wile, 1996. p. xv.

Chapter 3: My Teacher

We think that history is made up of the legends of giants. And maybe the shadows of the giants grow taller as the stories about them are told and retold. It might also be said that the shadows of these giants are filled with the forgotten stories of the people upon whose shoulders they stood, those whose stories were never told, those people who did not want their names to appear in the headlines or the marquees. Great contributions to Tai Chi — to any art — are sometimes made by people whose names have been forgotten. If many of those names are unknown to you, as well, you may prefer to think of the more local history. Of course, many of these are the sorts of folks who may have contributed considerably to the depth and breadth of the art, but their names might not be well known either. It's time to change that in one particular case.

Meeting Sifu

August 2015. It was a Tuesday morning very much like others that had come before. I found myself working out in the morning at the neighborhood recreation center. As often was the case, I was embraced in the ever-lovin' arms of my favorite treadmill and frankly...I was bored of it. Sometimes, if I got there early enough, I could watch a Tai Chi class. The teacher was an older fellow. He wore a goatee. He seemed somehow taller than he was.

My teacher is a very private man. And while he loves his students, and we are very loyal to him, I think he would rather avoid the attention of devils, trolls and casual gawkers. Plus, in the tradition of both the American mountain men and the Chinese Taoists alike,

Sifu has great respect and friendship for local law enforcement, but I think he would still rather avoid any imperial entanglements, so to speak. And I am pretty sure that even with the nickname, serious students will find him. They always seem to.

I had heard Sifu's name around Cincinnati in connection to Shaolin Kung Fu and Tai Chi. I had even tried to find him some years before. By then, I was four years into my studies in Tai Chi, and I had only scratched the surface. You know what they say about the teacher appearing when the student is ready. Apparently, the Cosmos must have believed that it was time for us to meet. On that particular Tuesday morning, I suddenly realized the obvious: they had a Tai Chi class right there. I inquired and the next time they met, a Thursday, I sat in. It took me at least a few minutes to decide that I really wanted to join the class, and within a few months, I knew that I was committed to studying with Sifu as long as I could, that it would become a central part of my life. I've never doubted my decision. I've never looked back.

He is a neighborhood fixture and has trained hundreds of students including military veterans and local law enforcement. He has studied with some of the greatest names in martial arts. "I've been lucky to train with some of the best," he has often said. "I didn't go looking for them. They've walked through my door." Lucky, indeed. I feel lucky to study with him.

The Old Powder Factory

There are venerated temples of martial arts around the world where generations of students pursue their journey of self-development, martial skills, or enlightenment through physical discipline. Such locations are sanctified over the course of history with traditions of their own. Imagine training at these places of mystery and manicured beauty. The floors, their patinas are indented by countless feet across untold years and then reverently swept pristine. Stone patios, matted training halls, and manicured gardens are hidden away by temple walls or mountain forests. Training hall floors are figuratively and literally stamped with disciplined footsteps on the journey to self-development or better understanding. The walls are adorned with the images of beloved teachers: sifus, teachers, masters from the past. Worn and well-used weapons are earnestly stowed on racks on the walls. These are the romantic idylls of magical places.

Closer to everyday local reality, martial arts can be practiced in whatever places are available and accessible: garages, living rooms, shop fronts on streets where the rent is cheap or in suburban strip malls, gardens behind the house, or the neighborhood recreation center or park. Many US martial arts studios feature window fronts or glass cases stuffed with trophies, displays of past victories and shadow boxes with brightly colored rank belts. Some of these studios pop up like mushrooms after a rainstorm and disappear equally quickly. Others become neighborhood institutions and last for decades.

The Old Powder Factory, might be an odd place to find expert instruction in the martial arts, but for years, you could. It is located on a hillside just north of Cincinnati above the shores of the Little Miami River. The concrete and rebar building complex was built in 1860 to produce ammunition: musket shot and cannon balls, perhaps in anticipation of the US Civil War. Either way, thanks in part to the Old Powder Factory, there were plenty of bullets.

The factory produced its last bullet or cannon shell in the middle of the twentieth century and was then abandoned. For decades after that, the site comprised run-down buildings, shattered windows, rebar, and industrial concrete. For years the increasingly dilapidated Powder Factory housed a warren of out-of-the-way shops for mechanical artisans and machine-shop engineers working on motorcycle engines or scrapping metal. It was something of a superfund cleanup site.

At night, locals say the site was, and still is, haunted. Someone filmed a low-budget horror movie there once. Someone else built an ad-hoc haunted house for Halloween one year—though I can't imagine that it took much effort to make it spookier than it already was. Adventure-seekers and scallywags, some armed, would sneak into the complex at night to catch their thrills and conduct sordid business.

The buildings had eyes, so they said. The police would show up far too quickly to apprehend trespassers and interlopers. The police always seemed to know. In the age of motion detectors, CCTV, and drones, that makes sense. However, for years stories were told about the security guard who patrolled the lonely buildings late at night with his favorite disciple, a giant German Shepard. You should talk to him sometime. He is my teacher, or Sifu. He might have a good story to tell you.

For years, Sifu kept a studio in one of the more intact buildings in back. The studio was outfitted with machine-shop heavy tools, ersatz living quarters, heavy bags, a speed bag, punching mitts, and martial arts weapons. There was a library of books related to martial arts. A picture of Bruce Lee hung on the wall. Other portraits of revered teachers hung on the walls, too. Such talismans had power.

As an aside, many years ago, I found myself at the Aikido Central Dojo in Tokyo, Japan. I was waiting for an early morning class to begin. On that particular morning, we students waited breathlessly for a particular treat: class that day would be taught by the master of the dojo, Ueshiba Kissomaru. Kissomaru was the son of the founder of Aikido, Ueshiba Morihei. As Kissomaru entered from the teachers' door, he glanced at the students who were neatly and patiently lined up on the matt. Then he glanced up at the portrait of his father, which hung front and center of the training hall. By then, Morihei had been deceased for many years. However, in that momentary glance, I could feel an exchange between the two. It was as though Kissomaru had an entire conversation with his father — perhaps about what he intended to teach that day. Then he began class.

The Training Hall

There is a veil through which some students are funneled from public studios, rec centers, and so on to more private training spaces, places where private lessons might be offered for advanced or invited students. In these places, advanced information is presented in carefully curated lessons to selected students. The Powder Factory was certainly that. But there was another location where Sifu taught private classes. He taught a Saturday morning class at his home. It was a yellow Cape Cod house in the suburbs. I asked if I could come and was invited. Later, he also began a Saturday class in Kempo Karate. I joined that as well.

The Saturday morning Tai Chi class comprised of some of the senior students, some of whom were teachers in their own right. They had been Sifu's students for many years. Some of them had studied with other teachers, and they came to Sifu because he has a particular style and a particular expertise. He has an intuitive grasp of Tai Chi and how it fits into the greater martial arts world. The classes at his house were private, and Sifu always seemed a little more at ease sharing the obscure details of the art. We fondly referred to these lessons as "the secret stuff," and it was comfortably meant for private ears. Some of it might be thought secret because many people who teach Tai Chi simply don't possess that information or understanding. It was information gathered from Sifu's five decades of martial arts study, practice, and contemplation.

In the spring of 2019, the owner of the house where Sifu lived decided to sell the property. Sifu was told to move out by the end of summer. He decided, despite offers and objections from his students, to move into a construction trailer at the Powder Factory.

By that time, the leaves on trees were beginning to change. The construction trailer had no heat or running water. Electricity would be piped in at some point. Renovations had begun to transform the dilapidated building complex into apartments. Sifu was not concerned about the coming winter. Personally, I suspect this might have been his version of a remote mountain hut. He had lived at the Powder Factory before, and he seemed to be comfortable there. Sifu was still employed there as the security guard, and he had worked out a deal that would allow him to move into one of the apartments when it was ready. Today, Sifu still teaches. He can be found at the neighborhood rec center and at the Powder Factory on the weekends.

Chapter 4: **Teaching the Art**

First, teach your students to love the art.

My teacher learned from his teacher that sometimes the best way to answer to a student's question is to let them figure it out for themself. It helps to develop a student's curiosity. Sifu believes that when a student has to figure out his own answer, he tends to remember the lesson better. On the other hand, every once in a while, the student will take the question a little too far and write a book. My Teacher, I think I have figured it out.

What about you, dear reader: How do you know your teacher is any good? It's a fair question. Maybe it's the one question you really want to ask. How do you know if they know what they are talking about? How do you know if what they have to teach is real? Authentic? Useful? Your teacher will become someone with whom you will spend quite a lot of time. Any teacher worth their salt will perceive things in you that perhaps you don't yet know yourself. They will see things in you — potential, challenges, areas in need of development or adjustment. They will have a large role in developing your character and teasing out the potential of your best self. This is not necessarily unique to Tai Chi. The same could be said about the teacher of any discipline. Maybe you are studying to be a musician or an artist or a writer, and in those cases, you want your teacher to also be good, authentic, useful, and perceptive. However, our discussion here is about Tai Chi. How do you know if your teacher is any good?

With respect to teaching, there are three interrelated variables to consider, and we can imagine them as three points of a triangle. At the apex is the art itself. On another corner is the student. On the third is your teacher We need all three for a successful transmission of the art. There is also an addition factor involved.

But let's begin by asking your teacher that foundational question: What are you teaching? Are you teaching the art? Or are you teaching students? If your teacher emphasizes teaching the art, they have a message to transmit. They have something to say. They have collected wisdom and understanding that they would like to preserve and pass along to future generations. If they emphasize teaching students, then they are interested in the development of their students as people. One side is about preservation of the art and its transmission. The other is about human development. Of course, we need all three for either mission to be successful. One challenge, of course, becomes how to determine the quality, authenticity, and utility of the art. Another question is the one we just asked: How do you know if your teacher is any good? Then, of course, we want to ask about the student, but we will get to that in just a moment.

We can take look at the authenticity of a particular teacher by looking at the message that he wants to transmit. To explain how that works, let's digress into physics.

Entropy

Entropy is the measure of the diffusion of energy from fields of high concentration into areas where energy is less concentrated. The dispersion of energy represents the loss of potential for that energy to do work. It also represents randomness, disorder, or chaos because the lost energy escapes along whatever path is least resistant or most easily available, and it disappears without really doing anything at all. For example, a hot oven will warm your cold kitchen. So, while the kitchen becomes warm, it doesn't help cook your food. A microwave oven, on the other hand, has less entropy. You can test this by touching the door. It isn't hot. It is more energy efficient in the sense that more of its energy is focused on cooking your dinner. More of its energy is applied toward accomplishing its designated job. Less of it escapes.

So what does this have to do with teaching Tai Chi?

Entropy can be a useful metaphor for describing the transmission of the art across the generations from one teacher to a student, who may in turn become a teacher with their own students. One goal and the challenge is how to transmit an authentic message that is true to the art. So when we talk about the body of Tai Chi wisdom, skills, and traditions that stretches back centuries, we see that the work of teaching is the effective transmission of the art from one generation to the next. The energy represents the strength, clarity, and vitality — the authenticity — of the transmission of the art, the message. Entropy could metaphorically measure the bits that get lost along the way from one generation to the next: the loss of understanding, of details, of signal strength. The message gets garbled, and the details get whittled down. Eventually, there is an error in transmission. Details and information get lost. Maybe the teacher didn't transmit clearly. Maybe the student didn't receive the message properly or only received part of the message. Maybe the student stopped receiving all together. Maybe they think they've learned everything there is to learn and they are finished. Maybe that student has become a teacher and thinks there is nothing more to learn. What would that be like? Imagine what it would be like to study with a teacher who tells you they know everything and that they have nothing more to learn.

Maybe they are your potential teacher? In essence, over generations, it is possible that the quality of instruction diminishes, that information becomes lost, or that the path forward becomes less clear. This is why, at least in part, many wisdom traditions, religious scholars, martial arts teachers, and so on are very interested in the answer to that deceptively simple question: Who is your teacher?

The question of intellectual or artistic lineage becomes important. With respect to our discussion on entropy, it is important to know how far a teacher is from the source, how authentic their understanding, practice and teaching.

As we have seen, in the formative years of Tai Chi, the secrets of the art were legacies passed down through the family or clan or to trusted disciples. There was very little diffusion of information because the inheritor of the family legacy was expected to devote his life to preserving, protecting, and growing the art of Tai Chi. Each generation would eventually pass it along to the heir. Even today, there are still legacy heirs of various martial arts in general and Tai Chi in particular. These are people who can directly trace their lineage to the family clans going back many generations and have been named the official heirs of their tradition. As tangible evidence of this, as I mentioned, the Chen family today claims to still have the saber that Chen Wang Ting carried into battle many hundreds of years ago. It stands to reason that his legacy heirs still possess his teachings.

For most of us, that is not the case. Most of us don't have an ancient sword passed down from teacher to student. Most of us may not get that close to the source. Most of us will never get to study with a legacy heir. It is difficult to suppose that all of us, particularly in the West, even have a clear lineage. Having said that, your teacher's lineage is one indication of their authenticity. If your teacher is proud to tell you who their teacher is or was, that is one indication that the teaching they offer is closer to the source, closer to tradition.

In physics, entropy only moves in one direction. There is no negative or reverse entropy. Areas of highly concentrated heat or energy always diffuse or radiate to areas of less concentration. Your hot oven will never draw energy from the surrounding cooler kitchen and become hotter. It just doesn't work that way.

In Tai Chi, however, maybe it does. Sifu has often said that the aim of a good teacher, his aim, is to have his students surpass him. Of course, that's a pretty difficult proposition. It's a pretty high pinnacle to reach. My teacher already has a many-decades-long head start on us. Better yet, he is always engaged in learning more, trying to gain a deeper understanding of the art. So while he already has a considerable lead in flying time over his students, he is also always still moving forward.

Negative entropy. How do we make the signal stronger? How do we concentrate the energy of understanding Tai Chi? How does that work? And here is my point: a good teacher teaches their students how to keep learning, to engage with the art over a lifetime so that even if there is an error in transmission, the student will continue to collect and build understanding of the art. Sifu has also told us that if you want to be a good teacher, you must be willing to continue to learn. Indeed, a teacher should always be committed to learning more. Not only does he mean that a good teacher thinks about how to more clearly communicate his lessons, but also there is also always something more to learn about the art. He is willing to put aside his ego and learn from his students. Often, students will gain and develop insights that the teacher never considered before.

The story of Tai Chi suggests that the primary utility of the martial arts in ancient days was to battle rival clans or bandits, to gather fortune and glory, or even to train imperial guards. That's not completely wrong. Yang Chen Fu protected a lot of information from his imperial masters. He also adapted Tai Chi for an audience of his contemporaries by highlighting its health and well-being applications. To be sure, Tai Chi has evolved over the years. The methods for teaching it have evolved. However, the core principles and the traditions are still the same. They are still passed along. That is the value of the art.

Among other things, self-defense will always be a primary aspect of Tai Chi — I hope. I hope that Tai Chi instructors will always teach the martial arts applications that are readily apparent and encourage their students to tease out the hidden applications and meanings on their own. However, the nature of the battles has also evolved. Obviously, and not to be underestimated, much of street combat today in America involves very powerful firearms – reminiscent of life during the late Qing Dynasty, perhaps? Ever-more powerful firearms might leave one wondering about the utility of open-hand combat or fighting with archaic, close-quarters weapons; swords, staffs, knives, and so on. It might leave us to question why we should spend so much time learning Tai Chi.

The utility of the art has evolved over the years too. Tai Chi always has had much to teach us about our personal development. Like the I Ching , it has a way of confronting us with a reflection of ourselves. It was a way of showing us who we truly are and what we can truly become. Furthermore, Tai Chi still has much to teach us about ideas like remaining calm in the face of danger, situational awareness, and navigating our immediate environment quietly and efficiently. Today, many of the battles in which Tai Chi has been shown to be especially effective are against ourselves — against our own inner demons and our own contemporary dysfunction and dis-ease. These might include battles with a variety of chronic, debilitating physical and mental health disorders. Maybe they always have been there. Maybe today we simply have a better vocabulary for and understanding of these things than they did during the Chinese dynasties of the past.

At the same time, we students of the art still owe a great debt to the early innovators and teachers of Tai Chi. Certainly the elders of Tai Chi Chuan, the notables, and masters of the story were incredible martial artists, men who contributed greatly to our understanding of the art. For many of them, Tai Chi became an impassioned quest for understanding, personal development, or enlightenment. The genius of Tai Chi would be greatly diminished if we didn't remember and revere these early masters. Their insights and understanding are invaluable and irreplaceable. They have retained the traditions of the art and also helped to maintain its relevance in the contemporary world.

Certainly, Unbeatable Yang Lu Chan is unique within the broader story of Tai Chi. I cannot imagine there would be another like him any time soon. However, he was reputed to be a very difficult teacher and master, particularly with respect to his sons.[61] Sometimes a true

---

61 Liang, 1996.

genius in a given discipline has little patience for those who are less talented or less understanding. Perhaps that might be applicable to Yang Lu Chan. However, based on the available accounts of his teaching style, I'm not entirely sure that many students today would have the stomach or the stamina to long endure such a difficult and demanding means of instruction. Is that what I mean by entropy? Maybe. And so, if very few students are willing to seek the path of mastery, it might be suggested that the age of the masters has truly passed. And is the pursuit of mastery even necessary for all students? Is there value in simply enjoying the practice of the art and being satisfied?

Still, there is great work being done by the teachers and masters of our generation. Teaching methods have evolved. If this were not so, there would be no reason for additional works and books such as this one. Tai Chi today has survived the entropy and erosion that one might expect from the transmission of any body of knowledge handed down over the centuries precisely because it has evolved and because new understanding is being added. Indeed, it might be reasonably argued that as our understanding of Tai Chi has grown, that growth has helped it remain every bit as vital and vibrant today as it has ever been. Tai Chi has adapted to meet the needs of contemporary times while maintaining its fundamental traditions. This is the work of venerable teachers in every age.

We can show the transmission of Tai Chi as a unique and distinct body of knowledge. We can also show how that transmission has evolved over time. The storied names of Tai Chi masters — the names that appear over and over again — were all innovators in their time. We know their names precisely because they made Tai Chi relevant for the times during which they lived.

With respect to Tai Chi today, I have personally heard several elder teachers speak with great reverence, affection, respect, and more than a little awe of the teachers who came before them and who shaped their personalities, worldview and martial arts skill. I have certainly watched my teacher become nervous at the prospect of his elder teacher planning to visit and review all of us students. It is easy, perhaps, to imagine that these elder teachers lament with all humility and no small amount of irony that the age of the masters has faded with the passing of their own revered teachers. Of course, today's generation likewise speak of our elder teachers with great reverence, respect, affection, and more than a little awe. So yes. There may never be another Yang Lu Chan, Yang Chen Fu, or Cheng Man Ching. No, we may never again see masters as storied and tall in stature as they, but as long as we keep their stories alive, there will always be — I hope — students who aspire to be.

Your Teacher

Again, we return to the basic questions. What makes a good Tai Chi teacher? How do you know if the person standing before you is truly qualified to teach Tai Chi? How do you know if they are the right teacher for you?

You will want to sit in on a class or two. That should not present a problem. Watch what happens. Pay attention to the sense of the class. What sort of atmosphere is there? Sifu says that if you want to know how good your teacher is, look at their students. Not only might they have something to say, but also look at how the students present in class. What does their interaction with the teacher look like? What is your sense of the energy or atmosphere in the room? There is quite a bit of trust that goes back and forth between a student and teacher.

The student, of course, has to trust that what they are being taught is authentic and that what they are learning will work and will satisfy their needs. Work for what? That depends on the student's goals. Are they looking for a health and wellness regimen? Are they looking for a means of self-defense? Maybe they are interested in developing themselves or building their character. Or maybe they seek the power to crush their enemies beneath their boot heels and revel in the lamentations of their women. Maybe.

A perspective student should be clear about their intent. However, that bit about crushing your enemies beneath your boot heels might be a little dramatic. You will want to moderate and curate your expectations. Expect them to grow and change over time. The teacher has to trust that the student will develop their skill and responsibly safeguard the information they are being given.

Listen carefully to what your prospective teacher tells you. Listen to the words and phrases that they use. What kinds of expressions do they use in conversation? What is the focus of their lessons? These will tell you many things. To be clear, however, there is no wrong answer here. Some students may be more comfortable with less formality. Some students prefer or even need a disciplined and formal relationship with their teacher. Does the teacher require formal class rituals? Uniforms? Titles? Many do. This may suggest that such teachers might require formal relationships with their students. Many students may find comfort in the awe and mystery of their teacher, and they may feel comfortable being told exactly what is expected of them — what they need to do to get to where they wish to be.

Telling Stories

At breakfast this morning, Sifu told me stories about his teachers. He has studied a variety of martial arts with some of the greatest teachers of his generation. "I didn't go looking for them," he told me. "I've gotten lucky. They walked through my door." He told me the story of how one of his most important teachers literally walked through the door of his studio and watched him teach a class. I am not sure that all of us get that lucky.

A Different Story to Think About

I had a professor in graduate school who was very different from Sifu. When he told stories, anecdotes, and so on, he talked about having met a famous comic book artist. Once, he had met a famous movie star! His office was brightly decorated with comic book toys, posters, and memorabilia. He was indeed a colorful personality. He told dramatic stories about his internship as an orderly in a psych ward. However, there were never any anecdotes about his professional work experience. There were no stories that illustrated any sort of philosophy about life. He was teaching us to engage in a discipline about which he seemingly had no personal or professional stories to tell. He had his doctorate, but he didn't even share anecdotes about his own professors, good or bad. No stories about clients whom he had served. Sure, occasionally, there were stories about things that had happened to him, but very few stories about what he did. What kind of teacher do you think he was?

Sifu often tells stories about his teachers and his experiences. He talks about how this teacher or that one would scold him to fix his posture. Or to make his empty step quieter. He talks about his teacher's ever-present pipe and how that teacher liked to answer questions by asking another question because he liked to let students figure things out for themselves.

Sifu talks about his travels to China with his teacher. There, they met the masters of the Shaolin temple. Sifu tells the story about how they happened to be in China in 1999 when the United States bombed the Chinese embassy in Belgrade, Yugoslavia. Fearing retribution against Americans in China, their Chinese hosts insisted on coming to the Beijing hotel where they were holed up to protect them. The Shaolin masters trained with them on the roof of the hotel. Sifu talks fondly about his colleagues, friends, and training partners. All of these people are remembered in his stories. They are legends, all.

Between Sifu and that former professor of mine, one has a trove of relevant stories, wisdom, and experience to share. One apparently does not. Which one do you suppose we might learn more from? To be fair, that former professor did not possess what we might call the hoary beard of wisdom. He earned his doctorate and seemed to think he was finished learning. He didn't seem to possess much curiosity. I don't mean to disparage him unnecessarily, but I do mean to impress a point. My dear reader, this book is about Tai Chi. It could have been about something else if things had gone differently. Guess which teacher I found more inspiring, more authentic? Guess which one has a continuing influence on helping me to grow? And which one is better avoided. In essence, this book exists because of the inspiration I have received and continue to receive from Sifu. But the point is still valid: What does your teacher like to tell stories about? Listen to them.

One last thing. If your prospective teacher has a great deal for you — but only if you sign up today…if they talk more about payment plans, contracts, and discounts than they do about the art, listen to that too.

The Story of John

The other night, an older man and his wife came to class. John clearly had some balance issues, and he was favoring one side of his body over the other. Sifu asked a couple of us to work with them and a few others who were several months into their Tai Chi journey. After class, John told us that he was recovering from a broken neck, the result of a fall. This and here he was coming to Tai Chi. I hope he continues.

We had a conversation about him later that began like this: "Well, his problem is…" Yes, he did have challenges. People, all kinds of them, come to Tai Chi all the time. And if one is willing to come to class and do the work and maybe practice at home, then the challenge becomes shared by the instructor. How would a good instructor help a man like John to understand Tai Chi principles and learn how to move better?

I have taught Tai Chi to people with Parkinson's Disease at a local resource center called Parkinson Community Fitness. And I have a secret to tell you: I have learned every bit as much from them as I have taught them. Parkinson's Disease is a chronic, neuro-degenerative disease that affects both cognitive and motor function.

Even high-functioning people with Parkinson's may present with a characteristic tremor or a shuffling gait. For the purposes of our discussion, people with Parkinson's may have a difficult time with moving and balancing.

One of my colleagues is a man who long ago suffered an acute traumatic brain injury. His injury resulted in a basket of cognitive impairments and serious damage to the nerves in his extremities. He has now been studying Tai Chi for several years and credits the art with restoring his balance and motor sensory awareness in his hands and feet. He moves better with every passing day. We can all see the improvement — all of us who are in class with him. We might be tempted to suggest his story is unusual or anecdotal, that it's just one story. Yes. Maybe. A hundred years ago, Cheng Man Ching had a very similar story to tell. Remember when a wall fell on him as a kid? The anecdotal evidence is there. And even empirical evidence demonstrates that Tai Chi's reputation for helping people heal is well deserved. All that is required for this is that both student and teacher are willing to show up and do the work.

The point is that people come to Tai Chi with all sorts of challenges. In one way or another, many of them are seeking balance. If the student is willing to show up to class and do the work, then the question becomes simple: Is the instructor willing and able to take what they have been given and guide the student to move and balance better — whatever that means? That becomes the instructor's challenge. What I mean to suggest is that a good instructor will take responsibility for understanding the student's strengths and limitations. A good teacher will seek to build on the student's strengths and bolster their limitations.

Teachers Create Change

Given what I just said, here's a little irony. If you are serious about your Tai Chi, then you will want to remember one thing: whomever you choose to be your teacher will become someone who exerts a great deal of influence on how you see the world and how you navigate it. Will they teach you to be angry, domineering, and swaggering? Or will they teach you to be calm, humble, compassionate, and confident?

The teacher's job is to create change and growth in their students. If your studies over the long term don't lead you to see the world in a different way, and you might not see change right away, and that's OK, what are you doing? A good teacher has a way of holding up a mirror and reflecting areas we still need to work on. It matters less where a student is when they begin, what challenges they might have when they start. Whether they are "good" at Tai Chi or not doesn't matter. It matters more what they can learn, what they are willing to learn, and where they can go.

There are a few things to keep in mind about the transmission of Tai Chi. It's possible that a teacher may find themselves teaching their student everything the student will know concerning the art. It's also likely that the teacher won't teach a student everything the teacher knows.

Sifu says that a qualified instructor absolutely needs to have an understanding of the traditions and the art and also the skill to demonstrate what he is teaching. "Never ask a student to do what you can't," he told me at breakfast one day. And if you teach someone something, "They had better be able to rely on it if they need to." What he is really saying is that anyone who chooses to teach Tai Chi, or any martial art, is assuming a tremendous responsibility.

He also says that a commitment to being an instructor or a teacher is more than a recognition of progress or achievement. And this may perhaps be one of the most important lessons about teachers: being a teacher is a commitment to further study. A good teacher doesn't stop learning because they get a piece of paper on the wall and a shiny title. If someone wishes to teach, they must be willing to continue learning — indeed, they must be eager to continue learning.

In the world of martial arts, it goes without saying that students are always eager to learn more — new and exotic moves and methods, the "secret stuff." The information that comprises Tai Chi is a treasure. Every teacher should take careful responsibility for that information. However there are plenty of reasons why a teacher might be reluctant to pass along all the knowledge that they have.

In the old days, the secrets of Tai Chi were passed down through the family clans to male descendants and disciples. As I mentioned, daughters did not often learn the family legacy because such secrets were highly valued and every effort was made to keep them in the family. This did not really begin to change until the Chinese Republic Era and later. It was also not common to teach Tai Chi to non-Chinese students until well later than that. We might not think of these as particularly good points of view today. However, viewed through the historical context of the times, there were reasons for those attitudes.

Today, a good teacher should take responsibility for what they pass along. If the student misuses or abuses that information, it is partly the responsibility of the teacher. Sifu believes a good teacher must know who it is they are teaching. "I'm handing you a weapon," Sifu often tells us. "I need to know you won't misuse it." He wants make sure we understand the responsibility of what he is teaching.

All of Sifu's students understand that if we misuse the skills he is teaching us, he will get wind of it. If he does, he tells us, he will show up on our door to have words with us. I always felt comforted by this. He is looking out for us. To me, this shows great respect for the art and for his students. I believe he would, too — get wind of it, I mean, if we misbehaved. And he would also show up and demand an explanation. I can't imagine that would be a happy conversation to have.

Teaching students

A good teacher always carefully considers and constructs the message of their lesson so that it is as clear as possible. However, doing so does not guarantee that the student will receive it clearly or understand it as it is intended. A lesson might be perfectly clear to the teacher, and the student still might not completely grasp the meaning. There is a fine balance between a teacher's efforts to ensure they are transmitting the correct message and the student's efforts to try to understand. A good teacher will carefully monitor their student's progress, perhaps by watching them carefully in class or by asking them open questions. A teacher might ask one student to explain the concept to other students. Asking a student to explain something to others will reveal gaps in their understanding. However, it will also lead them to greater understanding.

A good teacher only passes along information that the student is ready for, that they are capable of understanding. Students are always eager to learn new, and possibly more exotic, techniques and methods. That doesn't mean that they are ready for them, or that they have even mastered what they have already been given. It is often said that students want the secrets but they are less eager to practice what they have.

A good teacher cares very deeply about their students. Actually, Sifu says that a good teacher will always be grateful for their students. Without students, you cannot teach. An attitude of gratitude is a good place to begin. But it's more than that. More than that, there must be a lot of trust between student and teacher. To be effective, sometimes, a teacher has to be critical. Sometimes, they have to reveal difficult truths. Sometimes, they have to say difficult things that a student doesn't like to hear. It's part of the teaching process. Respect and trust are essential parts. A good teacher will take responsibility for the student's development. They must understand each of their students and adapt their lessons to meet the students' needs. Students are always eager for new information. However, a good teacher knows how to balance the flow of information so that each student gets what they need but aren't flooded with too much detail or information that is too advanced for them.

Students shouldn't be flooded with new things before they have mastered what they already have. And I don't mind telling you that this is one of my own challenges. Sometimes, I bounce around trying to learn and experience everything I can before mastering what I already have. Sometimes, I get distracted by some shiny piece of new information, and I get all spastic about chasing it down. Then I want to chew on it until it makes sense. On the other hand, if that wasn't part of my personality, this book you are holding probably wouldn't exist.

A good teacher doesn't need to "prove" anything to their students. There is no ego involved. Allow me to clarify that. A good teacher will be happy to prove their qualifications. Of course. But they don't need to stroke their ego. The point of teaching is to serve and to learn. It's about humility and not about building their own self-worth.

Your teacher might, however, from time to time, demonstrate what is possible; the light ahead, what is achievable. They might model what a student might hope to become with time and diligent practice. Among people who have acquired true mastery in any discipline, there seems to be a sense of confidence and humility. Think about it this way: Someone who truly understands the art knows that teaching is not about them. It's not about proving anything; it's never about dominating their students. A teacher should be able to demonstrate mastery, and while mastery is absolutely deserving of respect, the first sign of mastery of the art is mastery over the fragile ego. A good teacher is humble enough to acknowledge that they might make mistakes from time to time. No one is perfect. If they were, they probably wouldn't be any fun, and they certainly would not need Tai Chi. No.

A good teacher is even willing to lose sometimes in order to teach their students, to let them learn. Willingness to lose. A good teacher must to be willing to lose, or else they are setting limits on their students. Their best wish is for their students to surpass them. This is something that Sifu says often.

A good teacher respects the art, and they take it very seriously. They are committed to teaching the art and presenting authentic Tai Chi. These teachers are immensely important because they defend authentic Tai Chi — including the lore and knowledge — against the forces of entropy and easy sales. These teachers are very concerned with preserving the art and passing it along to future generations. They may believe that the traditions, all of it, are meant for future students to discover and master. The traditions comprise a body of knowledge and understanding — a box of jewels - for each student to discover, learn, value, and protect. These traditions must be protected in their most pristine and authentic form so that future generations may access and learn from them, too.

The Story of Bill

A new student came to my class last week. Bill. We were talking about how to move our feet. He commented that there is a lot of information to keep track of. There is. Maybe I've given him too much, too big a bite to chew on all at once.

Bill came back to class today. I think he enjoys what we do. He said, "I hope you know that what you are asking us to do is difficult to learn." The whole class snickered as if Bill had somehow stumbled upon a great secret. They commented, "Yes. We all know that. We are very aware of that." Yes, Tai Chi is not something that is easy to learn in a class or two. I asked him to celebrate the awkwardness.

"Oh, you mean like laughing at pain?" Bill asked.

"Kind of," I said. "It's more like remembering this moment. You only get to come to your first Tai Chi class once, and you have already passed that milestone. Sorry for your luck." Then I remembered to add, "But if you feel any sort of pain in class, stop what you are doing and let me know."

But I've been thinking about what he said in the context of something that Sifu often says: "We aren't so much teaching you Tai Chi as we are teaching you how to move." Even setting aside the added challenges of having a movement disorder like Parkinson's Disease, Tai Chi strives to teach us how to move or operate our body in a new and more efficient way. People with Parkinson's, in particular, often battle what's called the Parkinson's shuffle. As the disorder progresses, they may lose awareness or coordination in one foot or the other. As a result, sometimes the affected foot may drag, which raises the risk of a stumble or fall. Tai Chi has an answer to this, of course: awareness of one's body. We have the empty step. Tai Chi aims to teach students, all students, to become more aware of their body and how it operates.

I was showing a move called Brush Knee in class today as part of the 8-step Form. I noticed that Bill was leaving his rear foot behind. In other words, as he rotated his body, he was not rotating his rear foot as well. Bill was all twisted around. One foot was pointed in the direction that he wanted to go, and the other foot was still pointed in the direction that he had come from. This is very common for new students, and it's even a habit that many more experienced people need to fix, too. It's a fairly easy thing to fix — if you point it out and work to change the habit.

I stopped the drill to demonstrate the difference, and I illustrated the problematic posture. I could feel the twist in my spine and a corresponding pull on the muscles on the insides of my thighs. It felt as though my body were being pulled in two different directions. It felt really uncomfortable. I asked the class to try it for themselves and asked them how they felt. Then I corrected them and asked them to compare the two positions. Feeling the problem is the beginning of understanding the movement. Fixing the habit will take time. Patience. That's what Tai Chi is all about.

Videos, a Note

A few words about learning Tai Chi from YouTube videos. Doing so is certainly convenient, particularly if you can not find a qualified teacher nearby. However, it also has its pitfalls and challenges. There are many videos versions of Tai Chi Chuan now. It's difficult to know which one to follow. Some of them are really good. Others, less so. My best advice is to follow the ones your teacher likes.

For a beginner — for almost anyone — if you can find a video about the specific form you are working on, I think you can learn the big movements, the gross motor movements. However, it's easier if you already know the poses, have someone to review them with you, or are already familiar with them. You can pick them out from the video and put them in to the matching sequence. I think it is difficult to learn the fine motor moves and details behind the moves from a video. If you already have a teacher, it may still be tempting to supplement what they teach with videos. Be careful. While there might be many excellent and well-qualified teachers making videos, any one of them might be teaching something slightly different from your teacher. It might be confusing for you.

Chapter 5: The Journey

Sometimes, we undertake a journey for reasons which we think we understand, but later it is revealed that the journey has taken us on a completely different path than we expected. Most of the time, we begin a journey eager to reach our destination. However, Tai Chi is a journey of no destination. That is perhaps one of the most difficult concepts to wrap your head around. The effort, the practice, becomes the journey.

Sifu has said many times that true progress in understanding Tai Chi takes place in the space between classes. Great discussions happen just before or after class; for example, on the way out to the parking lot after class. Yes. And the greatest understanding comes from practice at home. He has said many times that coming to class every week can only do so much to further one's understanding of Tai Chi. Of course, not every student will see the value of this or wishes to take their understanding of Tai Chi to that level and that is OK. But for those who do, practice at home is indispensable.

One of my Tai Chi colleagues is fond of comparing Tai Chi to scaling a mountain: Tai Chi is a long slow climb up a mountain. Once you think you have reached the peak, you can see from your vantage point that there is yet another mountain, one taller still to climb. I think that's a good thing. It means that there will always be new challenges, new things to learn.

I'm not sure if it might be discouraging for some folks to say that the journey of Tai Chi can be a lifelong pursuit. There will always be something new to learn and puzzle out. Many folks choose to make their Tai Chi journey much shorter. Of course that is fine, too.

Sifu has said on many occasions that the students who do the best in the long run are those who struggle at first with the material. They tend to stick with it longer and engage more deeply as they struggle to master the details. He believes that the students who tend to pick up Tai Chi and martial arts quickly tend to be those who burn bright and then burn out. They master initial lessons easily and apparently without much effort, but once they come to a challenge, they tend to not stay with it. Like the proverbial race between the hare and the tortoise, these students who tend to start off quickly and make progress, often soon tire of what has become easy for them. Tortoise students start off slowly. These students struggle to make forward progress, but they don't give up. They keep moving forward despite their challenges. These are the students, Sifu says, who tend to stick with the art and who in the end, find their way to mastery. I think there are many means of motivation and reasons for sticking around, but the point is valid.

What I mean to say is this: if you are a beginner and you struggle with Tai Chi or find it difficult, then rejoice! Remember—you only get to go to your first Tai Chi class once. You only suffer beginner's wobbles once. After that, you can never again go back to being a complete beginner. Is that a happy thought? That one need only suffer once through the awkwardness and uncertainty of their very first Tai Chi class? Or is it happier yet to think that the feeling of awkwardness and uncertainty already begins to diminish with the first empty step? Can you even know that unless you have already been there and think about it in retrospect? Once you step into a river, can you ever step into the same river again?

Cheng Man Ching's Tool Box

There are a few tools that you will want to carry along on your travels. Sometimes, the road will seem long and discouraging. There might be times when you are unclear about where you are going. You might not always see the progress you have made or the destination ahead. Master Cheng[62] offers a few tools to take with you with regards to Tai Chi practice: perseverance, greed, and patience.

Perseverance

Tai Chi is the journey of no destination. But if you are on such a journey of no destination, how will you know when you have gotten there? How will you know if you have arrived? Perhaps the idea of having a "destination" in any art is merely illusion, a lie. Maybe it's a trick to seduce you into aiming for a particular destination and once you have reached that, then giving up, no longer moving forward, no longer listening. So even if you cannot see your destination, keep going, keep moving forward, keep practicing.

Perhaps you might look around and see others in your class who are farther along the road than you are. Maybe they float through their form easily and gracefully. Maybe they never hesitate, stumble, or stagger. Maybe you wish you could do that, and right now, it is all you can do to remember which move comes next. What if you stumble on a move that requires better balance? What if you become frustrated because you cannot yet make your body do what other folks can apparently do so easily? It would be so embarrassing. Right? No. Keep moving forward.

In all things, be patient with yourself and with your progress. Remember that any mistake that you might make or frustration you might feel actually means that you are making forward progress. Yes. It's another riddle: use every mistake and setback as a lesson. It means you are moving forward. When you get to the point where it becomes easy for you, and you can no longer hear the lessons Tai Chi has to teach, it means you are truly stuck. It might be a good time to reassess your thinking.

---

62   Cheng, 1999.

Greed

Happily, for people who feel stuck, there is a simple mechanism for becoming unstuck. It's called greed — which, in this case is the drive to learn more. It's the natural tendency of every student to desire greater understanding and more wisdom. It's the mission of every teacher to moderate how much they give their student and to make sure the student masters what they already have before giving them more. There is a balance between patience and greed. Desire for greater understanding drives the learning process. Trying to eat too much all at once will give you a bellyache.

Tai Chi always has more to teach us. There are always additional forms to learn, hidden applications to ferret out, and additional Qi Gong sets. However, your form has its own secrets to teach you with respect to moving.

Secrets and wisdom your teacher might know. Do not be too eager to learn everything all at once. For example, there are many worthwhile Tai Chi forms you can learn. Don't worry too much about learning all of them or even many of them. Different forms have different lessons to offer. Every one seems to have its own character. Choose one to work on and master at a time. Think about this: it's far better to learn and truly master one form than to it is to pursue many forms without really understanding them.

Patience

This is a big one. Sifu has admonished me more than once: don't worry about getting there. Enjoy the journey. Don't focus so deeply on the destination that you lose sight of the treasures along the path. There is no destination in Tai Chi. There are, however, many side paths that may lead to nuggets of additional wisdom. There is no reason not to explore them as they appear. And don't become impatient with your progress. Learn one thing at a time and work on that.

Aspects of courage

There are many aspects and manifestations of courage. Likewise, there are many kinds of fear. Here are five that I've collected. I'll explain them with regards to Tai Chi. Some of them came from Master Cheng, Some of them came from Sifu. Some came from rather eccentric life experiences. They still apply to tai chi. Several of them, have been repeated to me from several sources and so it's time to pay attention and learn from them.

DO NOT FEAR BITTER WORK.

This is Master Cheng's phrase, and it is a case where the idiom needs better translation. Wile suggests that by "bitter work," Master Cheng meant "pain"[63] or discomfort. Do not fear discomfort. It may come from daily practice. It may come from sparring in practice. It may come from pushing too hard past your range of flexibility. I agree that Master Cheng was referring to the discomfort of training. In Tai Chi, like many disciplines, we are teaching our bodies new habits, new ways to move. As we might expect, our muscles may become stiff or sore. It's difficult. Experience this, and embrace this. It means progress.

Something else to consider: Tai Chi is not meant to be strenuous exercise. It's not always meant to raise your heart rate or strain your muscles. Tai Chi practice is most of the time meant to be soft and gentle. Expect most of the time to work at about seventy percent effort. Of course, sometimes, you may feel energetic and wish to practice at full tilt. Nothing wrong with that either.

More importantly, if you choose to walk along the Tai Chi path, you should not fear to do the work of daily practice. Sure, somedays, your daily practice might feel like an effort. There may be some days when you just don't feel like practicing. What would your daily practice be like if you thought of it as "bitter work"? What would your daily practice be like if you embraced it? Approach it with curiosity

---

63   Cheng, 1999.

and joy. This is a good think to consider, even if it is unlikely to be what Master Cheng meant by the phrase.

Injuries are different. Do not fear becoming injured. Remember, fear of falling increases your chance of suffering an injury by falling. However, if you do suffer an injury of any kind, that's damage to the body. Stop your practice and seek help.

When I was younger, I participated in a karate tournament and cracked a rib. The tournament was on a Saturday. The next day, Sunday, was a big training seminar. My sensei at the time wanted me to attend the Sunday practice, to train through the pain so to speak. We didn't know yet that my rib was cracked. It was painful and my breathing was strained – two hallmark indications of an injury to the ribs. (Yes, I know that now.) Needless to say, going to Sunday training was a bad idea. It's one thing to embrace pain as Master Cheng suggests. It's something else to train while injured and risk making it worse.

DO NOT FEAR DISCOMFORT

In today's world, comfort is a commodity. It is something we are taught to value, something we can buy and sell. Comfort, ease of use — they represent a time for rest. A luxury. Comfort is also an illusion.

There is nothing wrong with discomfort. Discomfort is often the engine we use to move ourselves forward. Discomfort is a point at which we can recognize our need for learning and self-development. Discomfort is the point in the journey where we can begin to see the road ahead. In fact, for many students, the first few classes in Tai Chi can be an uncomfortable, awkward experience. They may be surprised by how easy and graceful experienced students make Tai Chi look and how sophisticated the moves actually are. So the good news is this: everyone who practices Tai Chi — without exception — has survived their first class, that sense of uncomfortable awkwardness, and they have returned for more. They've gotten past the awkwardness of learning how to move in a Tai Chi fashion, and they've gotten better.

The bad news is this: you only get to go to your first Tai Chi class once. After that, the more often you go to class and the more often you practice, the more you will progress. And the sooner your discomfort will evaporate.

DO NOT FEAR LOSING

As a kid in school, nothing is worse than failing a class or losing a fight on the playground. OK, getting caught trying to change a failing mark on your report card might be worse. Losing a playground fight can be a difficult thing for a kid, too. But that's not the point.

We fear losing because we fear being seen as "a loser." We think of losing as a blow to fragile ego. We may already suspect that we are somehow not good enough and that losing just proves the point. Winning might be thought of as prevailing against everyone else. We may think that winning or being "the best" is the pinnacle of achievement. If we win, we might even get a coveted trophy or medal. For students and teachers alike, the idea of "losing" in Tai Chi means something different than elsewhere in the world. As an adult, failure is quite different. If you do not fail as an adult at least a few times, it means you aren't trying hard enough. It means you are comfortable and coasting.

To be sure, there are Tai Chi competitions for push hands and presentation of forms. These are great. They can be a lot of fun. They can teach us valuable lessons. In class, you might play push-hands games. In sword classes, you might have sword-play duels or sparring matches. Conceivably, you might also find yourself in a conflict, either verbal or physical. On those occasions, you might want rethink what "winning" and "losing" look like. Perhaps.

The point is this: If your goal is achievement, there is nothing quite like victory to show it. If your goal is to achieve wisdom and understanding, there is nothing quite like the sting of failure to encourage you to learn from your mistakes. In victory, you've achieved your goal. It might be thought that you can savor the moment or rest. In defeat, you have been shown what more there is still to learn. The only question is this: Are you willing to look at these lessons, puzzle them out? Are you willing to listen? Sometimes letting yourself "lose" will help your training partner learn. Sometimes, it will teach you, as well.

DO NOT FEAR FEROCITY.

Ferocity is intense emotion. It is energy. It can be scary. We can feel it. Understand it. By itself, it can't really hurt us. Not physically. Not unless there is a fist behind it. Here are three things to think about. Regardless of how angry your opponent may be, it doesn't change the considerations of conflict and combat. Biomechanics is still biomechanics. Range is still range. If your opponent is beyond effective range, he can rage and storm as much as he likes, but he still has to move closer before he can hit you. The move is the important moment. Also, a strike is still a strike. The rules of biomechanical advantage don't change just because your opponent is seriously pissed off.

Second, it might be possible to exploit your opponent's emotions. If they are in a state of rage, maybe you can lure them off balance. Maybe you can trick them into making a mistake, such as overextending their reach, for example. Also, rage means they aren't listening. They aren't connecting to you. They are broadcasting, but they aren't receiving. If they are not receiving, you can be deceiving.

Third, anger and rage are fantastic motivators. Strong emotions can energize the body and mask pain or the limitations of perceived weakness. If you allow fear to become anger, you can leverage it to your advantage. It can energize your body and intimidate your opponents. This is why some warriors like to access their rage. Better warriors seek to understand it. Just don't let it eat you. We'll add to this later.

Do not fear standing still

For many people, standing still can produce a source of anxiety. What are we supposed to be doing? I don't mean standing in Wuji — meditation or preparation to execute a form. Wuji, ironically, is doing something. Calming myself and slowing my breath is doing something. Preparing to move is doing something. Waiting for something to happen is doing something.

What I mean is standing still. I mean standing completely still. Not being the center of attention. Not checking my phone. Standing still. We may feel anxiety because we are not used to it. "What are we doing?" "Why aren't we moving?" "But we're not getting anywhere." We aren't used to this. We are taught that standing still is simply not productive. Our Western culture tells us that we must always be productive. We must be doing something. Time is money, after all. The implication is that we must use time — every single moment. Accomplish something.

However sometimes standing still — sometimes rest — prepares us to move again.

One Hundred Days of Tai Chi

At some point, years ago, Sifu challenged a bunch of us to the One Hundred Days of Tai Chi challenge. He said that in today's world, we often don't take five or six minutes out of the day to do something for ourselves. Why not spend a few minutes every day practicing Tai Chi?

The challenge is simple. All you have to do is this: Practice Tai Chi every day for a hundred days straight. If you miss a day for any reason, you start over. If you are sick, traveling, or whatever, you still have to do your practice. If the work day gets away from you and you have a dinner date, you still have to do your Tai Chi practice before the end of the day. It's a hundred days of every day. Either you get it done, or you start over. Going to class does not count. The length and content of the practice can be anything you like, as long as it is Tai Chi. You are only responsible to yourself to make sure that your daily efforts are satisfactory. You could do a five-minute quick practice. You could practice for hours. You could do a single form. You could work on any form. You may decide that Qi Gong is fair game. You decide for yourself what and how much to do on a day. But you must do something. It doesn't take long to realize that if you do a cheap, rushed, practice, no one will know. At least you can still say you did something. You do come to realize, however, that you are only cheating yourself.

I mulled the idea over for some time before I committed to it. Sifu told me that it took him more than two years to get through a hundred days straight because he kept missing a day and had to start over. Other students told stories of remembering at near midnight that they hadn't done their practice and so jumping out of bed to quickly get something done. Here is a taste of what it was like for me.

NOVEMBER 2018

I began my first round of the hundred days of Tai Chi challenge. I accepted the challenge with one addition. I recruited a few of my friends from class to do it with me. Every day, we would all check in by text to make sure that we kept each other accountable. I told Sifu about my strategy, and he suggested that we up the ante. If anyone of our group missed a day, then all of us would have to start over. I'm not sure that Sifu realized at the time that his change in the rules actually made things easier. No one wanted to be "that guy" who made every one else have to start over. Every one of us checked in every day by text. The group of us got through our hundred days challenge on the first try.

When we completed the challenge, we celebrated with ice cream. Others expressed interest in doing it, and so our numbers grew. Round two did not flow as easily as the first round, but no one cared. We were all looking at the big picture — to practice every day something that developed us personally. We still check in every day.

THE NEXT PIECE OF THE PUZZLE

We completed a second round of one hundred days of Tai Chi. Today, the group still checks in every day. We've added more people to the group. And I got two new pieces of the puzzle from Sifu. In the first round, we struggled to find a place to practice and a time to do it. We struggled to build the habit of daily practice. In the next round, he said that all of those challenges should have been solved. We worked through them in the first round. Sifu said that the next round would change the game yet again. Now, we could concentrate on taking that habit to the next level and work on the craft. Take habit, make it a ritual. Take the muscle memory, and use it to build a deeper connection, deeper meaning, and deeper practice. Deeper focus. Deeper spiritual meaning.

Daily Practice

With respect to daily Tai Chi practice, the question includes understanding the idea of doubt. What exactly is it that you are uncertain of? Do you have concerns about your own ability to remember your form? Do you have concerns about what to practice? What is that about? Tai Chi practice can be as simple as putting one (empty) step in front of the other. Tai Chi practice can be as simple as finding one particular pose (Brush Knee or Part the Wild Horse's Mane) and standing statically in that pose for as long as you can stand it. Or if you know the sequence called Grasping the Sparrow's Tail, maybe working on that could be your practice. The point is, do what you can or what you remember, then go to class and ask for help fixing or filling in the things you forgot.

Maybe you are feeling a little lazy or tired or off. If that is the case, start with a couple of minutes or even a couple of steps. See if getting yourself to move won't lead you to doing more than you thought you were motivated to do. Every time you make the choice to practice — even just a little — you are reinforcing the your will over your body and reinforcing the habit to conduct your practice.

The point is, choosing to take even one step when you are feeling like being lazy is one step forward to building the kind of habit that leads to daily practice and further understanding of yourself and of Tai Chi.

Sifu has suggested that sometimes, a good time to practice is when you are already tired. Or when you are already off balance. Those are the times when it is most difficult to begin your daily practice and they might hold the most powerful lessons. I'll just leave that there for you to consider. There have been many days after class or after daily practice, when I kept notes about my experiences. Here is a selection.

SOME DAYS, MY PRACTICE GOES LIKE THIS: 1

My mind is restless and distracted today. Tai Chi practice is always a good indicator of where my mind is. The practice requires prolonged, focused attention to get to the very slow, intentional, focused movement. Wherever my mind is while I practice, it shows. Distracted, restless, or calm, my practice reveals it plainly. That is interesting to me because that awareness allows me to modulate my mind. It's an opportunity to literally slow down and pay attention to my intention.

SOME DAYS, MY PRACTICE GOES LIKE THIS: 2

I focus restlessly on my form. I begin it and find that something feels a little off. My balance is wrong. My posture isn't what I would like it to be. A strike is not timed properly. So I start the form over. I might go over that form again and again. Each time, I move through the form until I get to a problem. I fix whatever point of detail and then start the form over. Sometimes, I might spend a half hour or more and never really come the conclusion of a form that should take only a couple of minutes to complete.

SOME DAYS, MY PRACTICE GOES LIKE THIS: 3

I choose one form and repeat it several times. I don't really care whether it is perfect. I just move through it. And then, again. The first time might be a little clunky. Each successive time, I find myself relaxing into it more and more. I think about it less and less. By the third or fourth time, I am flowing through it.

SOME DAYS, MY PRACTICE GOES LIKE THIS: 4

I remember something we worked on in class, some detail or point of polish that applied to a particular step. I work on that. Maybe it's something about Repulse Monkey or Cloud Hands. Or maybe it's some piece of footwork or posture that needs to be addressed and adjusted. I'll spend my time working on it. I might not get through a form at all.

SOME DAYS, MY PRACTICE GOES LIKE THIS: 5

I feel rushed or distracted. I don't have so much time for practice today. I'm thinking about something else. I burn through the shortest form — the 8-step form — a couple of times and call it a practice. Sometimes, I am not so focused and I move through the form without really paying attention. I don't really think about what I am doing. I don't have any intention. I move too fast. I just think about getting done. Can I be finished yet? I try to slow down. On those days, I forgive myself and promise not to have too many days like that.

SOME DAYS, MY PRACTICE GOES LIKE THIS: 6

When I begin, I feel distracted and I feel like burning through the 8-step form a couple of times and say that's it. As I move through it though, I become dissatisfied with my attitude or my effort or my intention or attention. I tell myself I'll just do a little bit more and try to make it better. I'll continue to work on it and maybe an hour later, I'll decide I am satisfied with my effort and smile.

SOME DAYS, MY PRACTICE GOES LIKE THIS: 7

I began my practice today in the early evening. It was chilly outside the air was brisk cold but fresh. It felt good to be outside moving. It felt good to be a little cold. The sunset calm peaceful on the back deck as usual. I began without warm up. I should have stretched at least a little. I began with standing meditation and felt myself calm. That state seemed easy to get into today. Then I began the Standard Beijing 24 Step Form. My first two moves were really good. They felt smooth and connected and on target. I felt calm and joyous and free floating. Then I thought about how calm and smooth my moves were today, and I stumbled on the third move. It was that very brief instant, that shift in my awareness from nothing to self-congratulations that caused me to stumble heroically.

SOME DAYS, MY PRACTICE GOES LIKE THIS: 8

Yes, practice may comprise of one particular form done a couple of times: rush through it quickly and be done. I suppose that counts for the hundred days. Actually, practices like that in my opinion count every bit. Better that than nothing — even if it leaves me feeling slightly guilty, somewhat like I've cheated. I feel slightly lazy perhaps. Sometimes it feels like I'm getting away with something, like I'm being dishonest with myself or with the others on my team. Not only are those feelings OK, I also think they can be helpful if they motivate me to do better tomorrow.

SOME DAYS, MY PRACTICE GOES LIKE THIS: 9

I work on one form over and over. Or I pick one sequence from a form to work on. I manage to tease out a little more understanding of the form or the moves. Tai Chi coyly reveals one of its mysteries to me. I understand a little better how to move.

TODAY

I don't have to prove anything to anyone. I don't have to demonstrate or compete with anyone. I don't have to be better than anyone. I don't have to perform. I don't even have to be particularly good at Tai Chi. It's liberating. The only real empirical measure of performance I need to meet, the only measure of success, is that I do something today. Since I'm the only real judge of my performance, I get to decide whether my practice today is good or valid or enough.

Even if I practice with my friends at the park, it's still just something I do for myself. My practice doesn't have to be brilliant. It doesn't have to be efficient or productive or even beautiful or graceful. It doesn't have to be any of the qualities by which we constantly judge each other. It just has to be. That's today. I love it.

In class, of course, we have teachers watching and helping us to improve, teachers who offer insight and guidance. They might offer suggestion for connecting forms or for ways to interpret each move. They might push us to improve or to learn more. That's what they are there for.

Of course, there are things in life that we do need to meet the approval of others, activities that are judged by the quality of the final product. There is competition in a wide variety of areas in life. Maybe competition provides us the external motivation to reach farther. But Tai Chi, at least for today, is not one of those activities. Instead Tai Chi today is a bubble in time and space: a castle, a haven, a refuge of joy in mind and movement.

Distraction

Novelist Joyce Carol Oates said that "distraction often wears the face of the person you love best."

In other words, maybe it is your spouse, significant other, partner, child, or favorite fur baby that will most likely lead you into distraction. That is every bit true for your personal Tai Chi practice as it is for writing or any daily practice. Distraction can also come from social media, telephone, television, concerns about work or play. Distraction can really come from just about anything. Of course, you know this. Of course, having small children at home can be a powerful distraction.

You need to set healthy boundaries. You need to make the decision to carve out the time for yourself and do your daily practice. Is it OK to turn off the phone for fifteen minutes or a half hour? Is it OK to ask the people you love best to leave you undisturbed or to have someone watch the kids while you conduct your practice? What happens to your self-image when you ask that? My guess is that you will still love them, but you will also feel empowered. Maybe?

Motivation

Suppose you decide that you really want to begin a daily Tai Chi practice. Suppose you make a decision and a commitment of some kind to pursue this journey. That's great! But it doesn't mean that the discipline will come easily. Let's look at motivation for a moment. Maybe you don't yet know the answer to the following questions, but I want to ask anyway:

- Why are you doing this?
- What do you hope to get out of your Tai Chi practice?
- How important is it to you?
- What would it be like in a year or two, if you abandoned your Tai Chi practice? Or worse, what would it be like if you never began it?
- What do you think your life will be like in a year or two if you have a regular Tai Chi practice?

Maybe you don't have answers for those questions yet. Maybe you will try Tai Chi and discover that it simply isn't your thing. That's OK.

There are, generally speaking, two different types of motivation: external motivation and internal motivation. External motivation is where you commit to something for reasons beyond yourself. Maybe you have a partner, a comrade, or a group who are depending on you. Maybe you know that someone important is watching you and has expectations of you. Maybe you need to prove yourself to someone. External motivation comes from outside yourself.

Internal motivation comes from within. It's a commitment to yourself that you will do a thing even when no one knows or no one is watching. You are doing it for yourself. Sometimes even a person who is very committed and determined to better habit building can benefit from a little help. Often we can use external motivation to help build habits until the internal motivation can take hold.

Chapter 6: **Basic Techniques**

The basic techniques described here are among the first lessons that new students should think about and practice. On one hand, they teach the unique character and flavor of Tai Chi. They also serve as foundational ideas for constructing a long-lasting personal practice. Rather than trying to master these techniques by reading about them, they are most easily introduced being demonstrated by your teacher. However, the more you practice them, the more secrets they will reveal to you. With respect to Grasping the Sparrow's Tail, for example, remember, there is more detail than was is presented here. This particular sequence is a good example to illustrate a few of the basic principles of Tai Chi that we will get to in a moment.

Empty Step

It's literally and figuratively the first step a student new to Tai Chi takes. Empty step. Empty step is a way to move so that your body weight is on one foot or the other most of the time. Empty step teaches you to transfer your weight from one foot to the other quietly and smoothly.

The idea is to sink your weight onto one foot. Extend the other, placing your heel first gently and quietly down on the ground. Keep your toes up. Then while you shift your weight onto the empty foot, execute whichever move you're heading into. Learning how to extend the heel of one foot quietly and put it down under control of the entire body is a foundational technique of Tai Chi.

Imagine stepping onto a surface that you know is going to be slippery: you keep all of your weight on one foot and reach out with the other to test the surface. At its most basic level, you don't commit your intent or your weight to your extended foot until you know it's safe to do so. With time, you can build the control and flexibility to drop your weight and extend your foot without any noise. Of course, empty step can be a step forward, a step to the side, or even a step behind. Meanwhile, the rest of the body, the torso, shoulders, head, and so on move quietly — without disturbance, without adjusting the rest of your body.

IMPORTANT POINTS TO REMEMBER

First, you'll initially sink your weight and extend the heel of one foot. How far forward should your foot go? It's not necessary to extend too far or exert yourself too much. The lower you sink your weight, the farther your extended foot will be able to reach and the longer your stance will be. However, the farther you reach, the more energetic your practice will become. A really long step is not necessary. A shorter step is fine. But make sure your step is wide enough to support you without wobbling from side to side. You will want to keep your feet about shoulder-width apart. Your step should be steady and it should leave you feeling steady in your stance. When you have reached the level. you will want to keep your hips level. Move them forward and back, twist them at the proper moment, but generally keep them at the same height. Also, when you step out and quietly place your heel on the ground with the toes up, the heel is on the ground because you want to pivot on your heel. Pivoting on your toes is the next best choice, but according to Tai Chi principles, it does not offer the same biomechanical advantage.

But remember this because it's important: You should only pivot on your heel or even your toe if that particular foot is light. In other words, do not try to turn your foot if your weight is on it. If you do, you could strain or damage your knee. All of your weight should be on one foot in order to turn the other. This is the way of Tai Chi. Do not try to pivot on or move the foot that is bearing your weight.

Keep in mind that the example given of extending the heel out in front and somewhat to the side is only one example of how you can move. The principles of empty step can be applied to moving in any direction: Forward, to the side, back, or simply getting out of the way. The point is to move intently and quietly.

Learning empty step offers a variety of lessons. To begin with, it is a slow intentional move. To do it correctly, especially at first, requires concentration. It requires a different way of thinking about moving, which, in a sense, is what Tai Chi is all about. Not only are we learning a different way to move, we also want to begin to connect the mind with our movements. Developing awareness of ourself and how we move becomes important. The idea behind empty step is to organize the way the body moves. While learning it, we are learning to pay attention to the entire body, even—and especially—the parts that we might think are not involved in empty step. Empty step only works if the entire body is engaged in one way or another. What are your hands doing? Your hips? What is going on in your mind? That is what we mean by organizing the entire body. When it comes to the organization of the body, mind, and spirit, organized movement—for example. empty step—is what makes the whole greater than the parts.

Here is one other note about empty step. Sifu often says that empty step means moving quietly. He says we need that sense of moving quietly in order to better listen to our opponent or our environment. According to Sifu, understanding empty step is 80 or 90 percent of understanding Tai Chi.

Standing Meditation

It is called Holding the Ball, or sometimes Three Circles Qi Gong, Wuji Stance, or, Standing Qi Gong. Standing still. What ever you call it, one of the treasures of Tai Chi is the unification of mind, body, and spirit. Tai Chi develops this connection in ways other styles of movement simply cannot. It connects the mind with movement, and it offers an advantage over meditation and mindfulness practices because it involves the body and movement along with quieting the mind.

It is a kind of Qi Gong that appears to be very basic in its posture and practice. However, it takes more time to master the practice than the details. The posture is simple, really. Stand evenly weighted, both feet about shoulder-width apart. Feet are turned in somewhat. The knees are slightly bent but relaxed. The body is held upright. The shoulders are neither pulled back nor rolled forward too far. They are rolled far enough forward and the shoulder blades are spread enough to give the impression that the chest is hollow. The arms are held with the palms of the hands facing each other in a large circle as though you are standing inside a large barrel and are pushing outward with the arms, hands and back. The head is held erect, the back of the neck elongated, and the chin pulled in just a little. The hands are held palms toward each other and fingers spread but not touching, as though they are holding a ball between them. The belly is relaxed and allowed to expand with each inhalation. Draw breath into the belly, and let it expand. Let it contract gently on each exhale without force or tension. Everything is relaxed. Finally, allow the gaze to soften as you look between the fingers toward the distant floor. This is the posture of Three Circles Qi Gong, as my teacher taught me.

The first of the Three Circles refers to the feet turned in slightly, as though pigeon-toed. The second is represented by the hands holding a ball. The third is created by the arms and the back. What do we do with this? Quiet the mind and focus either on counting numbers or counting your breaths. In class, we customarily hold the posture and count to 108. Any number that is a multiple of nine is traditionally considered to be good fortune. However, sometimes, in my practice at home, I count a particular number of breaths or I set a timer. However, I have found that when the timer rings, I jump in surprise. It kind of ruins the calming aspect. It is enough to begin with a practice of five minutes or so. Eventually, you will want to extend your time. Some sources suggest that you work up to an hour. One of my colleagues stands everyday for an hour, however, I haven't gotten that far yet.

Clearly, Three Circles is a form of Qi Gong that focuses on the mind more than the body. However, there is still a strong physical component. Maintaining the proper pose means that on some level, attention must be paid to the body and to balance. Unlike other forms of meditation, you won't fall asleep.

What do we do with the mind? What to focus on while doing the exercise? There are variations, different ideas. Some include "finding" all of one's body parts, or checking in with them as you stand. Others include moving Qi energy throughout the body. At first, and for a long time, you can use your imagination to move Qi until you get to the point where you can feel it.

After some practice, you may begin to feel warmth or energy tingling in your hands. You may come to feel as though your hands are two same-pole magnets pushing each other apart. As you gaze between your fingers, you may be able to detect a subtle field between them. As you practice more, you may be able to draw this feeling into your arms. Perhaps it feels like pushing out as though you are pushing against the inside of a barrel. Perhaps it may feel as though you are activating the circle contained within your arms. As you practice yet more, maybe you can draw that sense of energy into your chest and direct it to fill your Dan Tien, the Qi energy reservoir located within your lower belly. This is the way Sifu teaches Three Circles Qi Gong. Of course, you may find other variations.

In all of them, the point is relatively the same: we can use this to learn how to sense Qi energy, then gather it, and then direct it throughout the body.

In fact, there is a practice called the Microcosmic Orbit. It is a form of active meditation that is designed to move Qi energy through a meridian circuit from the perineum up the spine to the top of the head and down again through the chin, throat, chest, and stomach, and then back to the perineum. There is quite a bit of detail that you can research and discover. However, in my opinion, begin with

Three Circles Qi Gong before you can make use of the Microcosmic Orbit exercise.

However, with respect to Three Circles, remember these points: First, learn to calm and still your mind. Watch the breath, but don't force it or hold it. For this exercise, breathe deeply and slowly into the belly, but there is no need for breathing to a count or holding the breath. It's enough to fill the belly and calm the mind.

Three Circles is a very simple but powerful exercise. It helps you to develop focus and concentration. We might suggest that it teaches you to quiet your mind, however, it does not. The point is not to quiet the mind. Instead, we want to learn to listen to the mind. We want to learn how to separate out the noise and distractions from awareness – from that still small voice of intuition.

The challenge of the exercise is similar to the challenge of any meditation exercise. You will feel distraction, monkey mind, and you will feel resistance. Your body will try to get you to stop early. It's a common phenomenon. The mind gets restless or distracted. These are natural feelings. In time, you will overcome them and improve your powers of focus, concentration, and calm.

A Few Moves: Peng, Lu, Ji, An — or Grasping the Sparrow's Tail

Before we go much farther afield, let's be clear about what we mean by poses and moves. Each pose is a stopped moment in the corresponding move. It represents the completion or full expression of the move. If we were taking a still photograph of Tai Chi, the pose is that moment when the moving parts of the body have all come to a stop in their proper positions. In each pose, we want to pay attention to posture, structure, weightedness, and so on. By "move," I mean the moving into the pose, its completion, and moving through the pose into the transition beyond. That is, by move, I mean moving through the spaces between each pose.

Many of the classic texts describe early Tai Chi as being comprised of eight poses (corresponding to the eight bagua, which represent the gates or trigrams of the I Ching) and five directions (each corresponding to one of five elements). These are the 13 original moves of Tai Chi. Of the eight poses, four of them form a sequence called "Grasping the Sparrow's Tail." These are Ward Off (called Peng), Rollback (Lu), Press (Ji), and Push (An). And many of the texts even suggest that if you understand Grasping the Sparrow's Tail, you will easily grasp many other Tai Chi moves.

As we become familiar with each of these poses and learn how to move, there are a number of questions we might wish to consider: What do you feel in your body when you make this move? What are the principles of Tai Chi movement that this move emphasizes? Of course, we will get to principles in just a bit. What are the martial arts applications? When I was first learning the moves, Sifu suggested that when you find the pose properly, correctly, it just feels good. This is a pretty subtle point, and perhaps we might not completely understand until later when we understand the proper posture and structure. But the question speaks to something very important. Learn to pay close attention to how your body feels, which parts are moving and how they move. Your body will tell you what you want to know.

From understanding each posture, we come to study the move into and out of it. Ultimately, we want to learn how to move in a Tai Chi fashion. What does this move have to teach me about the art with respect to how to move better, more quietly, and with greater efficiency? We already talked about empty step. We have to be single weighted before we can move a foot. If you are already single weighted, maybe you only need to move your non-weighted foot. Or, if you are double weighted, maybe you first need to shift your weight onto one foot so you can move the other. Another move might be more useful in exploring how to better move from the hips. Another one yet might illustrate keeping one's head up.

We want to think about the martial arts applications. Sifu always emphasizes the importance of this. Learn the martial arts applications of the various Tai Chi moves—or at least some of the elementary ones. Even if – especially if – you are not interested in learning how to "fight", learning the applications helps you to better understand the mechanics of the move itself. For example, it helps you to better understand how to – and why – rotate your wrist for a better strike, how to turn your hips while you shift weight from one foot to the other, or how to sink your weight at the moment of impact.

Sifu says that without an understanding of the martial arts applications, you are leaving behind the essence and treasure of Tai Chi. Without that side of Tai Chi, you won't understand the finer details. If you don't understand the applications, you might as well be waving your arms around or dancing, Sifu says. You won't fully understand how the change in your posture, waist, or wrist can change your entire structure. Learning the martial arts applications involves learning about biomechanics, how your body can be made to move more efficiently. To be clear, I am not suggesting that a student of Tai Chi must become a fighter. Not at all. I am suggesting that there is a wealth of understanding that comes along with exploring the martial arts applications of Tai Chi.

Having said that, most moves in Tai Chi have clear and obvious applications. For example, Ward Off (Peng), which is the first move in Grasping the Sparrow's Tail sequence, is easily understood as a strike. That is the most obvious application and the one commonly demonstrated with the pose. You might be tempted to ask what other applications you can find. The easy answer to that question, at least for me, is that the more you play with the move and the more times you ask that question, the more answers you can find for yourself. Let me offer you a clue, one that will add a completely new dimension to your thinking. Many times you can find interesting applications in the transitions between moves or by combining consecutive moves. This will require you to learn the sequence of moves and pull them apart. But the effort will be well worth your while.

If we think about the martial arts applications of these moves, the Grasping the Sparrow's Tail sequence has many lessons to teach us. First and foremost, taken in sequence, Sparrow's Tail teaches us to shift our weight between one foot and the other. Almost always in Tai Chi, your weight should be almost completely on one foot or the other. Sparrow's Tail teaches us to shift between one foot and the other. As we move through this sequence, indeed, as we move through all Tai Chi forms, we should be aware of how we are weighted.

Next, Sparrow's Tail teaches us the range of our strikes. At first glance, Ward Off and Press appear very similar. The most obvious difference is that Ward Off uses one hand to strike, and Press is also a strike but it uses the edge of one palm to support the other wrist.

Ward Off and Press are both inspired by a sense of expansion of the body. Something else to note: Ward Off is a one-handed strike. I like to view it as though the shoulders and hips are turned just a little. With Press, because both hands are engaged, the shoulders and hips are directly facing the opponent. This means that both strikes could have slightly different ranges. Ward Off might reach just a bit further, though it is most often close. Press needs to be a very short strike. Both make use of the hips in ways that are subtly different. If you learn both of these moves and play with them, you will see what I mean. You can learn the range of your strikes —whether they are too close to the body and collapsed or overextended and possibly taking you off balance.

Block

Block is not something we often use in Tai Chi. Block implies a sense of stiffness and muscular tension. However, we can use the idea of blocking to better understand the concepts of redirect and dissolve which we might use in Tai Chi. So let's take a moment to look at a block. In old-school, hard styles of martial arts, every beginning student is taught how to block a punch or a kick as a measure of defense. The lesson is either directly stated or implied that often a block against an incoming strike is meant to be hard, a collision of sorts. You are throwing an arm out to bash away the incoming strike. The idea is almost to cause pain or damage to the striking limb. You can damage it, disable it, or dissuade the attacker from using it to strike again. The end result is that, depending on the execution of the block and the incoming strike, one or both people will feel the impact. It will hurt.

A block often results in needing another block, particularly if your opponent understands the idea of combinations—for example, if they throw one punch, then another, and then another. A block may create an opening for you to launch your own strike. A block might be used as a sort of attack on the striking limb. You may wish to use a heavy or aggressive block to "bash" the arm of the incoming punch, for example. I've also seen guys break their arms trying to block an incoming front kick. In those cases, I don't think they were doing it right.

Redirect/Deflect

Redirect is the second strategy for responding to a strike. The best defense against a strike is to make sure that it lands anywhere but the target. Do this either by moving the target out of the way or by changing the path of the incoming strike so that it misses. Redirect means changing the path of the strike so that it misses. Redirect is not a hard block. Redirect is much softer. You can use it to distract the opponent's attention, steal their balance, or manipulate their structure. If you push the attacking limb out of the way with enough intent, you can change the direction of your opponent's attention. With enough of a sharp push, you can manipulate your opponent and distort the stability of his stance — attack his structure. Essentially, you can take his balance. If your opponent is off balance, then they can do nothing effectively until they regain it.

Dissolve

Imagine punching a cloud. You think you are striking at a large mass, and just as you think you are about to impact that mass, it dissolves. Your hand passes through it as though it isn't there. Dissolve is like that. Clearly, though, we are not clouds. We are physical people, and no one really wants to get tagged or punched.

Dissolve is one of the foundational concepts of Tai Chi. We can best understand it by comparing it to block and redirect though it is far from either of those. It means responding to the incoming strike with a sense of greeting and gently, calmly, softly moving both it and yourself so that the strike does not land where it is supposed to. You are simply not there. Let your opponent think they are about to land their punch, but at the last minute, they miss. You only have to change the path of the strike just enough so that they miss. And if you do it correctly, they might not understand why they missed. Dissolve, done correctly, means that you seem to vanish. Your opponent strikes, but they strike nothing. It is a means by which you manipulate your opponent so softly that they don't even notice until it's too late. Dissolve means reading your opponent but not allowing him to read you. It means knowing your opponent but not allowing him to know you. A really good dissolve can trick your opponent into overextending or overreaching so that they lose their balance or structure. You can use dissolve to draw in your opponent, to let them think they are winning. Let them close the distance. Then launch your own strike at close range or take their space. Dissolve is not quite the same thing as a boxer bobbing and weaving. A really good dissolve can make you seem to disappear.

To understand dissolve properly, you need to understand a few basic ideas. First, dissolve is about receiving the attack, greeting it. We aren't blocking it. We aren't even deflecting it. I don't mean "wearing" it or letting yourself get hit. We're talking about self-defense, after all, not self-sacrifice. To dissolve, be as soft as you can, and greet and "guide" the incoming strike. You want to connect so gently and softly that your opponent doesn't realize it. This does not require strength at all. Just the opposite: to be effective, you have to turn off your strength. Be soft and quiet. Be a ghost. Allow your opponent to think they are winning and that they are about to tag you—until they miss. If you use strength, your opponent will notice, and they will change their strike. Dissolve is what's meant by using four ounces of strength to move a thousand pounds.

This is just a representational list of basic techniques. Any of these could easily be included in the most important parts of your practice. It is plenty to get you started. Expect them to feel awkward at first. You might feel self conscious or resistance to them at first. As you build your practice, they will become easier. As you become more familiar with them, you will want to begin to add some of the principles in your practice.

Chapter 7: **Core Principles**

What makes Tai Chi distinct, what gives it its unique style and flavor, are the principles which guide the movement. While every teacher and master might describe their list of basic principles in their own words, the ideas are fairly consistent. You might also notice all of the concepts are interrelated. Yes, there is plenty of overlap between each of them. Balance is related to structure. Structure impacts breathing, and so on. The entire list of common, core principles leads up to three ideas, three concepts that make Tai Chi unique: move quietly, be organized in your movement and thinking, and energy expression.

And you might say, well, that sounds like a short list. However, each one has quite a lot of moving parts. So in order to understand each one, we first need to understand the foundation upon which these are built.

Rooted and Grounded

Simply put, rooted and grounded both mean being connected to the Earth. They are related to balance, structure, and movement. With respect to Tai Chi, rooted is related to structure and balance. Grounded adds an energetic or Qi component.

Rooted comes first. We don't often think too much about keeping ourselves upright and vertical. However, we can leverage our connection to the Earth. Just as a tree extends its roots into the ground, so too do we sometimes need to attach our feet to terra firma.

From a metaphorical point of view, the idea finds its roots, so to speak, in phrases that we use every day: "I'm down to earth" or "I feel grounded" or "I need to get back to my roots." In one way or another, these speak to being reoriented to one's self and one's surroundings, regaining one's footing or balance, or regaining an understanding of one's place in the reality of the universe or one's essential nature. Being connected to the earth means having a firm sense of self. In conflict of any kind, we must never surrender our identity. If we lose our footing, then we lose balance and fall.

From a self-defense perspective, being rooted is a matter of possessing functional balance and proper structure. Being rooted allows us to accept a certain amount of kinetic energy from our opponent without losing balance. We can make use of body mechanics and structure to direct that kinetic energy down to the ground or to the side. This is more than just pushing incoming energy downward or sideways. Rooted means connecting through the body down to the feet. There is also an attendant sense of dropping one's body weight through the feet also. The idea is to bend your knees and lower your center of gravity from the chest and shoulders to the hips.

It should be noted that rooting can only absorb and redirect so much incoming kinetic energy. But, according to Sifu, learning how to do so is an early milestone in one's Tai Chi journey.

Once rooting is understood and the skill becomes available, one can learn how to be grounded as well. Grounded is a more advanced concept than rooted and makes use of Qi energy in addition to mechanical or kinetic energy. The idea is similar, however. With grounding, we can learn to accept the expression of Qi energy from our opponent or environment and direct that to the ground. And, of course, the reverse is true, as well. One can also bring Qi energy up from the ground and use it for a strike or to move. Think of grounding like a lightening rod. Lightning rod safely ground or direct the energy into the earth. Lightning is far too powerful a thing for most trees to absorb, even ones with deep roots. It destroys them.

With grounding, one can direct incoming energy down or bring it up again to express it. In order to understand and make use of grounding, however, you have to understand how to sense and direct Qi energy. This is much more subtle. It takes longer to understand. It is also more powerful.

The Song of Tai Chi

Song is the mindful or intentional relaxation or release of muscular tension within the body and limbs. In a sense, Song allows the elbows to become bendy and the arms to become soft. Song does not mean letting go of structure or form and soft does not mean becoming weak or wishywashy. We still want to maintain structure and so on. Instead, Song promotes awareness of structure and form and allows you to improve them. It means receiving kinetic energy for the purpose of moving it out of the way.

Song is like being a sapling. You are still firmly connected and you have strong roots. You are connected to the Earth, even if you are weighted on one foot. Yet, the top of the sapling; the upper branches and trunk, is supple and flexible. It can bend in the wind and is still ready to release energy and spring back into its preferred shape. Song is the sense of being ready to receive conflict, gather energy, and to release it instantly according to the requirements of the moment.

Another useful metaphor for explaining Song compares the limbs to water hoses. As the water flows through them, they extend but they do not become stiff. As the water pressure decreases, they become softer. The idea is to keep enough water pressure in the hose to allow your limbs to move. Then, time the impact of your strike with turning up the water pressure. At the point when your strike impacts, reduce the water pressure again so you can move. When you are receiving a strike, begin with low water pressure so that you can move fast and so that your opponent does not sense your intent. Then increase the water pressure so that you can dissolve your opponent's energy or redirect their strike. The point is that there is no stiffness in a water hose.

Being calm allows us to move quietly, to listen to ourself, and to connect with ourself, others, or the environment. If you listen while you move, maybe you can feel the pull on your knee as you move without properly aligning your foot or maybe you can feel the wobble in your foot as you balance or move. Feeling these and other messages from your body can help you correct your posture, structure, and moves.

By contrast, if your muscles are tense, clenched, tight, your movement and reaction time slows. Your ability to move efficiently or generate power in your moves are also inhibited. For example, if you tighten the muscles of your arm while throwing a punch, you will activate the muscles that "push" the fist out, the triceps, as well as the ones that "pull" on your fist the biceps. Can you see how that will slow down your strike? The key is to be relaxed.

Without Song, connection with your opponent or with your environment is not possible. Without connection to your opponent, there is no dissolve; there is no sense of greeting incoming strikes. There is no sense of soft control of the situation. Anxiety, anger, fear, or eagerness take control. Without Song, connection with your opponent tends to become little more than an attempt at anticipating their intent or moves. This paves the way for misunderstanding or failure to achieve our desired results.

Single Weighted

The idea of single weighted teaches us to be ready to move without having to shift our body weight. Having to take the weight off of one foot before we can move adds an extra step. It slows us down. There are a few common expressions of this. If we are caught off guard, we might say: "I was caught flat footed". The simile of being like "a deer caught in the headlights" suggests being double weighted and worse, having to decide which way to move in the face of oncoming danger.

In Tai Chi, most of the time, you want to be single weighted. One foot is full: All or most of your weight is on the full foot. The other foot is empty: It has no weight or very little weight. You should be able to move your empty foot without adjusting your body, structure, or balance. That is the point. The empty foot is not committed. It is free to move or kick without a shift in your structure. The price for that flexibility is that the other foot must be firmly rooted. It must be fully weighted. In a sense, much of the time, Tai Chi is done standing on one foot.

Being double weighted means your weight is distributed across both feet. With respect to Tai Chi, there are very few instances when you want to be double weighted. Being double weighted can provide powerful structure, particularly if you are well rooted and grounded. The cost, though is mobility.

Timing

There is at least one very good reason why learning the martial arts applications of Tai Chi is so important, even if you have no interest in learning to fight. It introduces you to the idea of timing. If you are only interested in Tai Chi for its health and well-being benefits, you may not ever learn the importance of timing. Is timing important? Well, yeah. If you really want to connect with someone, you have to be on time.

Timing is not what you might think. Yes, you want your strike to meet its target at the precise point in space and time. However, there is more to it. The idea is simple. In executing a move, all of your various body parts move in different directions at different speeds. Every part of you must end up at the conclusion of its movement at exactly the same moment. In every move, the roots are in the feet, the hips drive, and the move is expressed through the hands. They all have to complete their movement at the same moment. Otherwise, your strike won't execute properly. You won't express as much power. Your move won't be quiet.

Why is all of this important if you aren't interested in learning to fight? Without attention to timing, you will never learn to be precise and organized in your movement. If you don't care about precision, you will never engage in listening to yourself. Timing requires precision. Precision requires self-awareness. A sense of timing requires self awareness. Learning timing is not an easy task.

Expansive Moves:
Your Working Space, Your Boundaries

In classical Yang Style Tai Chi, all the moves are meant to be large and expansive. In other Tai Chi styles, the moves might be small and compact. In classical Yang Style, the idea is to make a circle with your arms as though you were hugging a large tree. Make the circle as big as you can make it without compromising your structure; without over-reaching or overextending. Take up space. You deserve it.

Anything within that space, Sifu says, is your working space. Your goal, he says is to control everything within that space. And, of course, we want to control as much working space as we can. It's our bubble, after all, our space. At first thought, we may wish to keep our opponent out of our working space. We might think we want push them away and create distance. There are certainly times for doing that.

On the other hand, we may draw our opponent into our working space for our advantage. We might allow our opponent into our working space to capture and control a limb, steal their balance, or manipulate them to our own advantage. However, this requires an understanding of our own structure and it requires connecting with or finding our opponent.

There is something else to note about expansion. From a non-combat oriented point of view, expansive movements allow us to develop flexibility and test our range of motion. Expansion of movement also helps us to better understand structure, balance, and how to coordinate disparate, discrete body parts into moving with common purpose. Expansion-oriented moves help us to learn how to move with grace and flexibility.

Particularly as we get older, our tendons, ligaments, and fascia all stiffen, and our range of motion becomes limited. The only way to combat this creeping stiffness is to work diligently on retaining our flexibility and range of motion. Of course, there are many ways to do this. Tai Chi is but one. However, Tai Chi happens to be the discussion at hand. If you are more interested in yoga, I'm sure there are many excellent books on the topic. But this is not one of them. Either way, maintaining flexibility in the connective tissue (the fascia) helps us to maintain vitality and open Qi energy pathways through the body.

With respect to being expansive in your Tai Chi moves, you must also understand contraction. We might expand to ward off our opponent. We may expand into our opponent's space to take their structure or balance. We may expand to greet an attack and then contract in order to dissolve it. We might also contract in order to draw our opponent in close and then expand into a strike.

There's something else to note about contraction. If you contract too far, then your ability to expand again may diminish. Generally speaking, our bodies are constructed in such a way that our ability to generate force—a push, for example—grows and diminishes according to where our hands are in relationship to our shoulders and core. If our hands are too close to our chest, we have less force to generate a forward push. Generally speaking, we are at the apex of our biomechanical advantage to push when our hands are in front of our center and our elbows are somewhat bent but not overextended.

If you find yourself too contracted, you still have a couple of options. Instead of pushing, you can dissolve. Instead of moving your hands, you could move your body away from them. You could try moving your hands in circles. This is something to play with and explore.

Lastly, there are plenty of small-frame styles of Tai Chi available. These make use of smaller, more compact moves. They can be beautiful and very effective styles. I can only speak about Classical Yang style, which is known as a large frame or big-move style. However, if we understand how the big expansive movements work, then we can certainly understand and adapt the smaller and more concise movements as we need.

Stillness is the Mother of Movement

Have you ever seen a cat pounce? Or a snake strike? In each case, before moving, the cat or the snake's entire body is calm and coiled. When it launches its strike, the whole body explodes from stillness to action. There is no hesitation. There is only the whole body moving. Like a spring releasing. There is no single part of the cat or the snake moving by itself. Everything moves as one coordinated whole.

Sometimes you will see a house cat sort of wiggle as it prepares to pounce. Likewise, before throwing a punch, often you will see someone drawing their fist back, winding up, or tensing. You might even see them pulling their body back into a "ready" position. If they begin double weighted—with their weight centered across both feet—they must shift their weight onto one foot or "rock" before they can move forward. All of these things are noise. None are stillness. All of them need to be eliminated from your habits.

Don't even seek to find calm, balance, or single weightedness. Instead, be calm and balanced. Launch your strike from wherever your hands are. From wherever your weight is, launch forward with your entire body into your strike.

Balance and Listening

THE HUNTER[64]

There is an old story told about an ancient hunter who was out looking for something to make his evening meal. He stopped in the

---

64   Adapted from Opie, Parabola, 2007.

reeds by a lake to drink some water and to see what sort of game he might find there. He saw an egret perched on a branch. It was close enough for his spear. Quietly, slowly, the hunter raised his spear about to strike. Then something caught his attention. The egret was focused on something and was itself about to strike. The hunter followed its gaze and found it was stalking a frog. The hunter watched. The frog, in turn, was hunting a large bug. It too, was hungry. And that large bug was sneaking up on a smaller bug. The hunter imagined that that smaller bug was stalking some creature that was smaller yet and that smaller creature was stalking its own prey. How far down it did go? The hunter could only guess. Suddenly, the hunter looked over his shoulder at the sky. He threw down his spear and ran away.

The next two concepts, balance and listening, have several dimensions to them. So for example, with respect to balance, we might at first think that it only applies to physical balance. However, balance can apply to aspects of the body, mind, and spirit. Listening, as well. Of course, it means physically listening; however, there is also a more subjective sense of turning in.

BALANCE

Balance in all things is perhaps one of the greatest treasures of Tai Chi. Empty step, moving quietly, and being rooted all require it. It is the key to moving efficiently. You will need to master these ideas in order to progress in your Tai Chi studies.

When we talk about balance, there are two variations. There is standing on one foot. Let's call this functional balance. If you slip, stumble, trip, or kick, how fast can you recover your equilibrium? Even if you do fall, your sense of balance in the moment can affect whether you get hurt.

The second kind of balance is less situational and more wholistic. Wholistic balance refers to a general sense of calm and awareness that you carry with you throughout your day. It's not that you don't experience emotions or mental disturbances. You do, but you understand it through the lens of Wuji, the Void. You may "wobble" or "stumble" emotionally, but you quickly regain your composure. I find that the study of one teaches the lessons of the other. Stay tuned. We'll get to those in a moment.

Functional balance

Functional balance is more physical. It's about balancing in the moment. Keeping yourself from physically falling over. First, it's important to recognize when you are standing on one foot which foot is actually doing all of the work. The foot on the ground—the stabilizing foot—is working hard; the lifted foot should be light and floating.

What do you do if you can't (yet) stand on one foot? If your balance is horrible?

First, balancing is a skill that you can develop. Depending on how well your skill is developed, you might have to work a little harder. That's OK. You might begin by using a table or chair to support yourself while you practice. Over time...hopefully...if you work at it, you may find that you need the support less and less. If you are unable to balance on one foot, you can also try shifting all of your weight to one foot and simply raising the other heel. Keep that toe on the ground for stabilization and support.

There are a couple of tricks and realizations that can make this just a little bit more easy and authentic. One idea is to imagine that your weighted foot is very heavy. Imagine it is made of iron or stone and push it into the ground like ballast on a ship or boat. Use the weight to keep you upright. Become rooted. As we discussed, imagine that your weighted foot has roots growing down into the ground that anchor you there. It is helpful, I find, to sink one's weight into the foot on the ground. Bend that knee, and allow your weight to sink into the grounded foot. This is the root of rootedness.

Be calm of mind and focused. Set these imaginings clearly in your mind. Doing so crowds out uncertainty and instability. There is no room in your mind to both imagine something and allow yourself to wobble. Note that the "wobbling," the instable impulse, will try to capture your attention. When it does, you will lose your balance. If you are nervous or distracted, you will find the work of being balanced on one foot to be very difficult. Indeed, standing on one foot can be an appropriate test for how relaxed and focused you are.

A very powerful idea is to imagine that your center of gravity is in your Dan Tien which is one of the reservoirs of Qi energy in the body. The Dan Tien is located a couple of inches below and behind your navel. When we talk about sinking your Qi to your Dan Tien, it has the effect, imaginary at first, perhaps, of lowering your center of gravity from your shoulders to your belly. It helps to activate your core and helps to drive your movements from your waist instead of from your shoulders.

The lesson of using your imagination to find your balance is helpful, I believe, because the implied lesson is that you can use your concentration to crowd out any intrusive thoughts. The harder you concentrate on imagining roots growing out of the bottom of your foot and sinking into the ground and the more steadfast you are about it, the less likely that intrusive or distracting thoughts will distract you from your purpose.

Eventually, however, you will find that you no longer need to rely on these imaginary constructs and that rooting the weighted foot will become second nature, and your sense of balance will improve. Of course, that comes with practice. It's a good thing that you won't have to think about these forever because you will find that with Tai Chi, there are plenty of other things to think about and to train your body and mind to do.

As an aside, if you are practiced and comfortable with lowering your center of gravity, then if you were to lose your balance and fall, you would not fall as far. And if your knees are already bent in the instance of a fall, then simply bend them further and guide yourself to the ground. A higher center of gravity is harder to balance. A lower center of gravity is easier to control.

LISTENING

Another important value of Tai Chi is to develop skills of listening with a sense of curiosity instead of judgement: Listen intuitively to yourself, listen your opponent, and listen to your environment. We talk about moving quietly. Listening and moving quietly are imprecise metaphors. Yes, we want to learn how to move without sound, to learn how to walk softly. More precisely, this means learning to move efficiently, precisely, and intentionally. Tai Chi seeks to scrape away, to polish the burrs and spurs of unnecessary, uncoordinated, disorganized movement or expressions that betray your intent. There is — or should be — no expenditure of unnecessary or disorganized energy.

Tai Chi wants to teach you to pay attention to what's going on in your body and in your mind. On a small scale, we also want to polish away any unneeded facial expressions — a grimace or twitch — that telegraphs our next move. Any muscular contractions — tightening of muscles —that contradicts or restricts our intended motion is noise. When throwing a punch, for example, relax. Don't to tighten your biceps. Simply put, biceps are meant for pulling things toward you. Throwing a punch, obviously, is pushing away. These two muscle motions contradict each other. This is also "noisy," and it reduces the power and effect of your punch. Granted, in Tai Chi class, we don't always punch things. But the idea is absolutely applicable in other ways we move. Another example is stepping forward from standing still. If you have to shift your weight from one foot to the other in order to step forward, that is also "noise."

On a more subtle note, we can even ask where our energy is. Where our minds are. Are they united, calm, and focused to a common point and purpose? Or are they distracted and pulled in different directions? Is it the person standing in front of you? Or is it something else and this person just happens to be a convenient target? If you are in a mood to react harshly or stringently, if you are cranky or angry, ask yourself what it is you are really upset about.

Master that. It's important. Once you learn how to pay attention to that, you will want to expand your listening to your opponent. How do they present energetically? What is their intent? Where is their focus? What is their next move? Is their mind and energy calm? Are they focused? Or are they defused and distracted? Are they hesitant or resolved? If you are in an argument, very likely, they have a point that they really want you to acknowledge. They want to be heard. Metaphorically speaking, being heard might just mean they want to impress their point, but if hearing their point means a punch in the nose, you might want to get advance notice so you can avoid it.

Now, can you shift your own attention from the noise of your fear of your predicament to what is going on with your opponent? Can you set aside the noise that your own emotional reaction is generating so that you can attend to circumstances effectively?

The next step for you is to expand your sense of listening to the environment around you. What is the ambience? What objects, challenges, people, or distractions are around you? Does your opponent have friends who might join the conflict? Making this a habitual exploration will require quite a bit of flying time — practice.

Listening is definitely something you can play with. Sifu says he often tries to sense how many people will be on an elevator before the door opens. You can also play with sensing how many people will be in a room or what their disposition will be before you enter.

THE MOUNTAINS LISTEN

Many years ago, I travelled through China because I was on my way home from Japan. I had joined a collection of eight or so travelers from Europe, and the US. We travelled by bus together through the mountains to a small town called Yangchou. The bus dropped us off at an intersection in the middle of the night. We stood in a circle with our bags piled in the center. There was a very light rain. We were getting wet and we didn't really know where to go. Between the darkness, the glare of street lights, the rain, and the fog, it was quiet and kind of creepy. There was no one else on the streets. We had reservations at a nearby hostel, but we didn't know exactly where it was. It was an age before cell phones had been invented, and none of us had ever been to that town before. As we stood there in a circle, talking about what to do, suddenly it got very quiet. Conversation died. Our eyes adjusted to the darkness and to our surroundings. The dragon's tooth mountains quietly appeared out of the gloom and darkness. These steep, sharp mountains, are like teeth, and they circle the town. They were famous in that particular region of China. They appeared quietly and suddenly. They were giants that had snuck up on us in the dark and circled us. They sat quietly on their haunches and listened to our conversation. It was a moment of awe.

NOISE

What are you listening for? Noise can be more than simply noise. Any disharmony in your movement can be considered noise. Maybe you have a wobble in your step, a momentary hesitation or uncertainty, the dip of one shoulder, or the turn of a hip. It could be a sharp gaze at your target. Any of one of these or others might telegraph your intention.

Detecting "noise" in your opponent and quieting the same in yourself can help you to win fights. Listening or paying attention to your opponent's posture can tell you quite a lot about him and his strategy. At the same time, Tai Chi wants to teach you to move quietly so that your opponent doesn't "hear" you. This is the idea of the maxim "Know your opponent, but do not let him know you."

The Story of the Snake

Today, I was thinking about the snake from the classic story. In class Sifu had us play push hands (Tuisho). Push hands is an exercise meant to simulate a sort of highly stylized sparring. The idea is to develop sensitivity and softness. At its most basic level, the game is to touch the back of your wrist to your partner's. You move your hand with theirs in a variety of patterns, always keeping contact. You should not press against your partner's wrist too hard. The feeling should be like having a butterfly trapped between your wrist and theirs. Don't let it escape but don't squash it. Be soft but firm. Practice moving your hand with theirs in one of a variety of circular patterns. But your hand doesn't move on its own. It is coordinated by, connected to, and driven by your hips.

So why the snake? Imagine a rattlesnake for a moment. It coils its body in preparation to strike. One part of its body is rooted firmly on the ground. When it launches its strike, its whole body moves with coordinated purpose. From its belly and tail, it pushes against the ground and launches its head forward, fangs first. Until it launches its strike, the snake's body is soft, connected to the ground or rooted, and it is completely calm. It is not tensed at all. That is what we are trying to learn. To move like a snake. Circles, coils, softness, all of it.

Chapter 8: **Forms, The Book of Tai Chi**

With respect to Tai Chi, a form is a standardized sequence of postures or moves. In karate, a "kata" is the same thing. In yoga, it's the same idea is called a "flow". The Tai Chi form is, among other things, the primary means of transmitting the study of Tai Chi from teacher to student. There are many forms, and different forms have different provenances. That is, you can trace the history of a form and to it came from. Of course, the farther back in history you can trace a form, the longer its provenance, the more authentic it is thought to be. Every form seems to have its own character and energy, as well. For example, Sifu has a favorite form called Dr. Wu's 24-step Form. Another form I practice often is the Beijing Standard Yang Style 24-step form, which was created by the Beijing National Athletic Commission in 1956.

We've talked in these pages quite a lot about various books written about Tai Chi. Remember one (more) thing: Tai Chi was created and crystalized during times when many people did not read. Even as late as the late Qing Dynasty or even later, during the Chinese Republic Era of China and later, many people were illiterate. Until Yang Chen Fu, the idea of picking up a book to learn Tai Chi would have been unthinkable because for many people the reading itself would have been more mysterious than the Tai Chi. Keep in mind that for much of the history of the world, reading has been viewed by the general public as a form of magic.

And yes, before mechanized printing was invented, handwritten scrolls had certainly been passed privately from teachers to trusted disciples for centuries. Many of these made use of poems, songs, and metaphors that could only be deciphered if you already knew what they meant. They were meant to safeguard family secrets and jog the master's memory while teaching. China did have a strong Confucian ethic that created a literate civil service. However, even with that, I imagine that literacy rates among the common people were probably low as they were anywhere else. And so the transmission of the techniques and principles of Tai Chi was done through the creation and repetition of sequences of moves; the forms.

It wasn't until almost the twentieth century that books became cheaply printed and widely distributed. It might be interesting to note that even many of the mass market Tai Chi books contained photographs and illustrations that were meant to guide the practitioner through whatever form was being described. Learning movement through static photographs is really difficult. The photos serve better as waypoints or markers to recall the sequence of moves, rather than as means to learning a new form.

In other words, the forms have always been the traditional means to transmit the core principles and ideas of Tai Chi. The "book of Tai Chi" is not the one you are currently holding in your hands. The book of Tai Chi, metaphorically speaking, is the form you study, whichever one that may be. "Reading" that book requires repetition and practice. It is a very tactile and experiential process. It requires moving. Read your book of Tai Chi over and over. (And, from the shameless plug department: Read this paper book about Tai Chi over and over again, too.) Allow yourself the space to understand that every time you practice, you might learn something new. There is ever more detail you can learn about your form. Much of it, you will learn as you go, if you let yourself be open to it. Each time you practice, your form may reveal to you some of its secrets. That is, if you listen. The form, whichever one you study, "is like a self-teaching encyclopedia of the science of movement, and of the martial arts techniques, and also of the correct use of breathing."[65]

---

65 Jou, 1991. p. 130.

As you practice various forms, they begin to reveal their character. For example the Beijing Standard 24-step form has, in my opinion, a taste of Confucian influence. It was designed to be commonly taught to the people and to be a sort of glue for the great society. It has something of a "civil service" nature about it. It presents sort of a homogenized Tai Chi that is appropriate and easy enough to teach many people. And while it has its martial arts applications, they are neatly hidden away. This particular form focuses on developing balance, structure, and expansive, organized moves. It is quite suitable for teaching beginners. It is a very refined and very popular form. And so it is also quite good for mainstreaming Tai Chi across society and for building community.

One of Sifu's favorites, Dr. Wu's 24-step form, on the other hand, has more of a Taoist flavor, at least in my opinion. Its provenance is shrouded in mystery. Sometimes I like to imagine that Sifu first learned it while on a retreat in the mountains. Though, he said he learned it in Southwest Ohio, where there are more highways than high peaks. Furthermore, Dr. Wu may refer to Dr. Fred Wu, who was a famous teacher there in the second half of the twentieth century. However, that is somewhat speculative and the form itself may be older than that. In any case, Dr. Wu's form is a great form. It is more pragmatic than pretty. It has a more individual, eccentric feel, and it seems somehow more rebellious. It feels more transformative for the individual. It does have its lessons to teach about the common principles; rooting, structure, timing, and so on. It also combines some moves that are clearly martial in nature with mysteries related to Qi energy cultivation and expression.

The Classical Yang 42-step Form combines elements from several of the major houses of Tai Chi. It was created so that each of the houses could participate in national competitions and feel represented. This, too, has a sense of building the great society. Nevertheless, the 42-step Form includes some common Yang Style moves found in the shorter forms and more complex moves that are not. Some of my colleagues do not prefer this form because it is longer. However, I find that the more I practice it, the more familiar it becomes and the shorter it seems. How much sense does that make?

Another form that is particularly popular is Master Cheng's 37-step form. This is the form that Cheng Mann Ching brought to the United States and to Taiwan.

There is also Yang Chen Fu's 108-step form. It may be the same or similar to the one that Chen Fu got from his grandfather. It is reputed to take as much as 20 minutes to move through and presents quite a lot of information to learn. There are still plenty of folks who learn and practice it.

We also have an 8-step form and a 16-step form. Each has a different flavor and different levels of complexity. Some forms are meant to have large, expansive moves, others small. Some forms conceal their martial arts applications. Others display them boldly. There are even secret, or Michuan, Yang-Style forms. These are described as small-frame or small move forms. When it comes to forms, of course, every teacher teaches their favorite one.

The Process of Learning

Your form. Your teacher will select the first form for you to learn. This will be based on what they have studied and what they think is appropriate for you. However, regardless of which one it might be, the process for learning it is the same.

You will begin by learning the gross motor moves. Your teacher may ask you to watch or follow along as they move through the form. You might begin by memorizing some of the poses. Either way, you will want to learn the sequence of poses. At first, this will be a slow, rote memorization of which foot goes where and which hand does what. In this phase, it is a laborious process of training your limbs to coordinate properly so that your body ends up in the right place. These are the big movements that you learn first.

When you have all of the poses memorized and can find each one without too much difficulty, then you can begin to learn how to transition from one pose to the next. Each pose will become a move. You will also begin to think about the empty step and polishing your moves. You will begin to look at the details — the fine motor moves. Empty step will put greater demands on your sense of balance.

One progress marker or waypoint in your understanding happens when you no longer need to think about how to move or what move comes next. You will be able to move through your form without hesitation, without pausing to remember what comes next or which foot goes where. You must be able to move through the form with proper structure and balance, but you must do so without thinking about proper structure and balance. As you progress, you will begin to incorporate structure, softness, expansion, timing, and breathing into your form. Then there are the finer details of each move to learn. As you progress past these landmarks, cognitive function moves from rote memorization to meditation.

Transitions: Moving from One Pose to the Next

When you can do that properly, you can begin to explore the spaces between the poses — the transitions. Part of making your Tai Chi efficient and effective is to understand how to move from one pose to the next. And yes, the transitions have meanings, too. They have utility and applications. The spaces between moves are useful. Eventually, you will come to learn that your form is something like a song — a silent graceful song. Each pose comprises a note, and like music, you will begin to think about the spaces between the notes. Each pose will become a move and you will begin to think about the tempo and transitions between the poses.

Of course, what we are aiming for is to move seamlessly from pose to pose until the poses are no longer there. Through practice, each individual move will melt into the one after and the one before it. It is very important to complete every move, to take it to its full extension. But we learn not to stop at that point. The form becomes one continuous move. Only then, can we "forget" the poses and flow through them. Only then, does the cognitive function switch from thinking to meditation. Think about waves on a beach. Every wave crashes on the sand and extends as far as it does and then recedes. The water never stops — even at the end of its reach. Every wave flows as far up the beach as it does and then recedes without pause and the next wave follows. It never stops. It just keep coming in waves. You can think of it as individual waves — individual poses. You can also think of it as the tide: a singular, continuous, rhythmic function of water, a complete form.

Learn the form to be able to move like waves on a beach. Only then, will the gross motor skills required to perform the form be complete. Only then, will the student be ready for what comes after.

THE FORM IS NOT TAI CHI

Having said all of that, are you ready for another riddle? In class today, Sifu talked about many things including the forms. "The form is not Tai Chi," he said. Then he gave me a stern look and added, "But don't write that down. It will get me into trouble."

When he said "me" he meant "you." He meant me; Brian. He meant, "If you write that down, YOU, Brian, will get into trouble."

I met his gaze and nodded. But in the back of my mind I was thinking: "My apologies, my Teacher, but I've already written that down."

"Beginning students won't understand what that means," he said. "You'll lose them."

The form is not Tai Chi. I've heard him say that many times. What does that even mean? The forms want to teach us how to move. Your form will train your body and mind to organize and move as one whole unit. It will teach you how to breathe and how to listen to yourself and your environment. As long as you pay attention to the core principles, it will teach you how to move quietly, efficiently, and with purpose. The form teaches us to understand ourselves.

BUT THE FORM IS NOT TAI CHI

I confess that I have not studied Master Cheng's form. However, there are a few clues in the story of Cheng Mann Ching that may be helpful for our understanding of Tai Chi in general. I wrestled these clues from the book Master Cheng's New Method of Tai Chi Self-Cultivation. The translator, Mark Hennessy, writes that in Cheng's form, there are 36 poses to correspond to each of the 36 trigrams—ideograms—represented in the I Ching .[66] He also added one more secret or left-handed technique. Cheng Man Ching, as we have learned, taught his 37-step form in the United States and Taiwan, and it has become very well known. He first introduced it in a book published in 1949. This was only a few years after he edited Yang Chen Fu's book, which described Chen Fu's 108-step form. Earlier, we asked why he would so dramatically alter the ideas of his teacher.

There is an additional mystery. In the foreword to the book, Hennessy writes that Master Cheng changed his form slightly from version to version. Hennessy commented that no reference has been found from Master Cheng as to why he did that. His form varied slightly over time, but it was always considered to have 37 poses. Hennessy says it's a mystery that he can speculate about but for which he can offer no definitive answer.

Maybe it's not that great of a mystery. Consider this. First, Tai Chi is a living art. It evolves slightly in every generation, with every new teacher. To be sure, there are fixed points in its storied history. As we mentioned, the Beijing National Athletic Committee standardized some of the forms in order to popularize and homogenize Tai Chi to help build a great society in a country that contained a wide variety of cultures. Of course, there can be little doubt that the powers in Beijing also sought to assert control over one of China's cultural treasures. However, even the details of those standardized forms

---

66 The number 36 is perhaps a nod to the traditions of the I Ching , the Book of Changes, which is the foundational thinking of Taoism, the indigenous spiritual philosophy/religion of China. The book is based on 36 Hexagrams. The 37 poses is a nod to that tradition: Thirty six postures, plus one secret or left-handed posture.

and the interpretations of the moves they present vary subtly among practitioners and teachers. One master turns a wrist this way, another that way. Every teacher has their own particular area of interest so it's no surprise that what they choose to emphasize in their class is as individual as they are. Having said that, there are still standardized forms, which invite common discussion and display across various local groups and traditions.

Not too long ago, I was having a discussion about Tai Chi with a shaman friend of mine who had happened to have learned that same Yang 24 Step form in his travels. We watched each other perform it. He noted that if the form is interesting to watch, that's because it is beautifully done. It was the same form done with a few minor stylistic differences. There were what amounts to accents on different syllables, but the form remained the same for each of us.

At the same time, Tai Chi evolves. Why did Master Cheng change his teacher's form? It is well documented that Cheng Man Ching created his 37-step form because he figured that many people would not have the patience or discipline to master and practice a form as long as 108 steps. This makes sense. Cheng Man Ching simply removed the redundant parts from the 108-step form. In our class, we spent almost a year learning the Yang Style 42-step form. That time spent did not include looking much at the fine detail – All of the fine detail came later still.

And why did Master Cheng change his own form over time? Who can say for certain. My guess is that the changes to his form represent changes in his understanding of the art. Perhaps he added or altered details to correspond to additional insights he gained over time. I like to think that it suggests that his learning of the art continued throughout his life. Over time, his thinking became deeper, perhaps more nuanced. He did not let his thinking become stale or calcified. He continued to learn — as every student should.

Compare that to this one more thought. It's an important one. Yes, Cheng Man Ching altered his teacher's form dramatically by publishing his own New Method just a few short years later. He shortened and changed the sequence of moves, yes. But he did not change the art. Remember just a couple of pages ago when Sifu said that the form is not the art? I think this is part of what he meant. I imagine that Master Cheng thought very deeply about Tai Chi. If you compare Yang Chen Fu's book to Master Cheng's,[67] you do see that the sequence of moves is different. But the basic techniques and the core concepts, the ones you just read about, govern how to move in Tai Chi and the philosophies behind them remain the same. In other words, Master Cheng changed the sequence of moves, but he didn't change the ideas that power them. He would write later that he wanted to remain true to the principles that Yang Chen Fu aught him.[68] It suggests that the true secrets, essence, or treasures of Tai Chi are comprised of these core concepts and not the particular sequence of moves. The form is not Tai Chi.

These foundational ideas and core concepts weren't really original with Yang Chen Fu either. He learned them from his father and uncle, who learned them from his grandfather Yang Lu Chan. Yang Lu Chan didn't invent them. He learned them from the Chen family. As we've seen, in every generation, the form changes for a variety of reasons, but the song remains the same.

So when my teacher says, "Practice your form every day, and the form is not Tai Chi," here is part of the reason why. The simple answer to Master Cheng's mystery of the 37 poses is that the story grows a beard, so to speak. It grew and changed as Master Cheng grew in his understanding, practice, and teaching. At the same time, we balance tradition and evolution in hopes of gaining understanding. In my own experience, that seems to be the way of Tai Chi.

---

67 Yang Chen Fu's book was first published in 1934. Cheng Man Ching first published his in 1935.

68 Cheng, 1985.

Chapter 9: The Five Energies

Many years ago, I had a conversation about Tai Chi with a student from another local school. He was trying to help me to understand the philosophy his school taught. I don't even remember his name, but I clearly remember the conversation. At his school, there was quite a bit of discussion about seeking immortality. I asked him what did that even mean. No one lives forever. How can you become immortal? His response was simple and profound: "I don't know much about living forever, but I will be immortal until the day I die."

What does that mean? With respect to Tai Chi, we come to think about developing vitality, balance, calmness, and agency. With respect to the Taoist roots of Tai Chi, immortality might simply come to mean maintaining vitality, agency, and clarity long into old age instead of suffering a long and painful decline. Maybe immortality simply means holding onto the vital and effective self for as long as we can. How do we do that? How do we maintain the vitality of the self? We do this through understanding and developing the five energies. These represent five different interwoven, interconnected aspects of the presentation of the self. Each is a mountain to climb and explore. In the following section, we will explore these in greater depth. For the moment, a few words of introduction are in order.

Different sources present the five energies in different orders. I prefer to present them in order from most corporeal, literally and figuratively, to the most abstract. In the development of one's understanding of each of these energies, the order that I have presented them seems to me to be the most pragmatic.

We will begin with developing our awareness of the physical aspects of Tai Chi—for example, the body. From there, we will move onto an awareness of the mind. I prefer to list the mind as the second energy, and maybe not everyone would agree with me. That is OK. Many people who are interested in self-awareness already have some level of understanding of what the mind is and how it works. It is worth building on a foundation of understanding that we already have before we move into the more uncharted territory of esoteric and abstract ideas relating to energy and spirit. Also, we want to invoke and develop the powers of concentration and imagination. The ability to concentrate means holding focus on a construct or idea long enough to make it effective — or to plant it, so to speak, and allow it to take seed and grow. Imagination also becomes a useful tool as well. We can use it to conceptualize abstractions so that we can develop them and develop awareness of them.

For example, if you are not yet at a level where you can sense, feel, or manipulate your Qi, you might need to develop concentration skills and it might be helpful at first to imagine what that is like. Yes, the doctrine of "fake it until you make it" is in play here. Here is why that works, at least in part. It is related to the mechanics of metaphysics. Imagination opens up acceptance to the possibility that abstractions exist. It is not enough to pay lip service to the idea that Qi exists, for example. You must ingest the idea and let it becomes part of you—so that it becomes instinctual. Only then will you be able to sense what is already there.

Another reason I like to put mind before the higher-level more abstract energies of Qi, Jin, and Shen is because I want to have a discussion about the emotions before we get into all of that. Emotions contain great energy. If you don't understand how they function or impact you, then you will find your efforts to understand the higher energy levels will be distracted or derailed entirely.

Note: We never want to tamp down, repress, or ignore our feelings. Doing so will lead to bad things manifesting inside you. At the same time, it is important to have at least a basic understanding and awareness of our feelings so that our emotions don't eat us. In essence, we need to get our mental house in order before we move on to more esoteric, energetic, and abstract spiritual concerns.

The third energy is Qi, and we must learn to sense our Qi or internal energy. We might think of Qi as the fuel that powers our stove or engine. After we learn to sense and cultivate our Qi, we can begin learn manipulate it or express it. That becomes Jing or Jin. From there, we move to an awareness of Spirit. Spirit, or Shen, is the most abstract and mysterious. Pretty much every source you read describes it differently and with good reason.

The development of each or any of these five energies represents positive progress. If all you get out of your Tai Chi practice, for example, is a better sense of physical balance and bodily movement, then congratulate yourself for a good practice and achievement that will serve you well. If you progress to the development of better concentration and cognitive functioning, better yet. If you come to understand how your body works and moves and you have successfully organized your mental and emotional furniture, you may find that would be enough for you. You may not wish to go farther. Congratulate yourself yet again. If you go even further, you have some great surprises in store.

Then there is this: maintain your progress. Every sharpened blade becomes rusty if you don't care for it. Don't allow your progress to melt away or let yourself slip back to where you began if you chose to stop or interrupt your practice. Always seek to sharpen your blade.

Also, Sifu is very careful to be clear with this warning. Generally aim to develop these in order. Begin with the body and progress to the mind. We might use the mind to assist and augment understanding the body, and that would be OK, but master those before moving on. It is tempting to skip ahead and go straight for Jedi powers — whatever that means. But unless you begin with the discipline and stability of the body and mind, not only will you never be able to pull the spaceship from the swamp, so to speak, but you might also run a serious risk of hindering your development or even setting yourself back.

Developing each of these five energies can help us to create an organized and effective self where the whole being is greater than the sum of each part. I cannot tell you whether developing all of these things will lead to enlightenment, immortality, or whatever. Remember my friend who aims to become immortal until the day he dies? I have not yet gotten that far. Not yet. Happily, I have yet to achieve either mortality or immortality.

Remember also, if you choose to walk down this path, you should expect to spend a number of long years developing your understanding of these. For now, remember that having a sense of our own physical body is the root of movement and the beginning of awareness of the self.

Chapter 10: **The Body**

Today in Class, We Were Cranes

Remember that old story about Chang San Feng? The one in which our hero realizes the secrets of Tai Chi by watching a sunrise battle between a snake and a crane? When I think about that story, I often wonder if the snake survived. Today in class at Parkinson's Community Fitness, though, we imagined ourselves as cranes.

Indeed, many of the Chinese martial arts find inspiration from watching various animals move and applying those insights to their martial arts practice. Common ones include tiger, monkey, bear, deer, and many others. There is even a crane style.

Why cranes? What could being a crane have to teach us? When a crane spreads its wings, it is not compact or closed in. The crane, or any bird, spreads its wings wide to catch the wind. When a crane spreads its wings, its moves are long, soft, and graceful. A crane is balanced and poised. Likewise, in Yang Style Tai Chi we want to move with a sense of expansion, with long, graceful moves. We want to have good structure and balance, and we want to take up space as well. Among other things, this helps us to understand the range of our reach. If you understand your range properly, you can choose to meet incoming strikes farther away from you or closer.

We also reviewed Grasping the Sparrow's Tail because, hey: bird motif! Grasping the Sparrow's Tail is a sequence that appears in many Yang Style forms. I wanted to play with the feeling of spreading our own wings and while keeping our heads upright. I wanted the students to feel a sense of expansion, to practice taking up space, making themselves big. The idea is to make big arm movements without overreaching. Your weight has to be squarely on the weighted foot, pressing down into the Earth. Your head is completely upright, and your shoulders are over your hips so that you aren't leaning over and off balance.

We added to the feeling of keeping the head properly upright and our shoulders relaxed and slightly rolled forward as though we were holding crane eggs in our armpits. This helps to keep everything soft and helps to keep those internal energy meridians open and flowing. Keeping that space in the armpits also reminds us to keep a slight bend in the elbows. We don't want to have our elbows locked out. That is not very graceful, and it is not Tai Chi. I told my class that for myself in particular, I must be mindful to keep my head and gaze up. I have an old habit of counting ants on the sidewalk while I move through my forms. This is something I continue to work to correct.

Learning to understand the body is the point at which all students of Tai Chi start. We want to learn to move in a precise, organized fashion and we want to remember to keep our balance and our breath at the same time. Proper posture or structure is of great importance. So let's begin with structure.

Structure

Chang San Feng writes: The energy of Tai Chi is drawn up from the Earth through the feet and legs. It is controlled by the waist., directed by the spine, and expressed through the hands and fingers[69].

Body structure, or posture, is really important in Tai Chi. Paying attention to our structure helps us to understand how to move better and how to balance ourselves. Tai Chi can help you to become aware of this. Here are a few things to think about.

One of the first lessons I learned in Tai Chi is that when you find the proper pose for a given move — the one where all of the different

69   Liao, T'ai Chi Classics: New translations of three essential texts, 1990, p. 89.

parts of the body are connected and in alignment—it just feels good. If you take a moment to find proper Brush Knee posture, for example, it will feel right. It's about structure, feeling solid, balanced.

Begin thinking of structure as the intersection of maintaining balance, body mechanics, and the ability to move or strike. Good structure corresponds to the idea of biomechanical advantage. Simply put, if you are on your feet and you are ready to move or strike, you have some level of structure. If you are off balance or feel like you need to adjust your body position before you can move or strike, your structure is broken. Understanding that requires understanding the form and functioning of the body.

Having good structure helps us to better understand our reach and range. If we are taking care to maintain proper posture then we will find that our arms can only reach so far without leaning forward toward the target. Leaning forward is an invitation to overextend. Reaching too far makes you vulnerable. You may be tricked into losing your balance. Overextension means that you have to recover before you can move again and that slows you down. Likewise, if we are collapsed in our movement, having an upright posture will show this to us, too.

Now, let's add to it. Good structure by itself has benefits to better health and functioning of the body. There is a significant health justification for keeping the head up.[70] Having a stooped, hunched posture can present negative effects on various body systems. Hunching over with the head canted forward, out of alignment with the shoulders, can put stress on the heart and lungs, and it can reduce lung capacity. It can pull the spine out of alignment causing compression of the thoracic and cervical vertebrae. Having a constantly hunched posture and compressed vertebrae can affect blood circulation and the nervous system. It may also restrict the spine's ability to twist or rotate. Also, restriction of air flow can cause

---

70   Tom Bisio is a practitioner of Tai Chi's sister art Xing Yi and a practioner of Traditional Chinese Medicine. He writes about how all of the systems in the body are interrelated.

problems with circulation in the extremities and may even affect cognitive functioning.

What would it mean to go through your day knowing that your brain did not get enough oxygen? How would it change your life if you did get enough oxygen to the brain? Poor posture can rob us of energy and make us sluggish and sleepy. Standing or sitting upright can be energizing and can help focus the mind.

Another common postural problem is that I often see is that people walk hunched forward. Sitting all day might cause tightness in the hamstrings, the hips, or lower back. Of course, all of these are connected. Being overweight or letting your belly spill forward, for example, can pull your spine out of alignment. Of course, these days, many people spend their time hunched over a computer or a cell phone. Remembering to straighten the posture periodically might undo some of the effects. The problem is that bad posture can affect your energy level. Long term, it can restrict your lung capacity and affect your heart health. It's a really bad way to move through your day. Practicing structure regularly as part of your Tai Chi practice might help you reverse the habit of poor posture.

HIPS

In Tai Chi, a great deal of emphasis is placed on learning how to move differently. We don't wish to step, then shift our weight, then turn our hips, then throw a punch. Instead, we wish to have the entire body move in coordinated, common purpose. I mentioned a moment ago that in Tai Chi, every move is rooted at the feet, driven by the waist, and expressed by the hands. It might seem counterintuitive, but the expression of the hands is the least important part. If you have proper footwork and the rotation of your hips, then you can strike effectively with your elbows or even with your shoulders. Of course, that affects your range, too.

Let the turning of the hips drive empty step, shifting the weight and the impact of the strike on its target. No movement is wasted, and every move is driven from the waist. This is the second aspect of sinking your Qi to your lower Dan Tien, your lower Qi energy reservoir. It has the effect of allowing you to focus on moving from your waist instead of from your shoulders. Don't allow your butt to stick out or stay behind. Don't let your belly fall forward. Instead, stay upright, tuck the pelvis in, and drive with the hips instead of leaving them behind.

Something else to think about. If you allow your waist to be the governor of your movement, then you are less likely to hunch over, less likely to drop your head, and less likely to drive from the shoulders. Driving from the shoulders limits the power of your strikes, tends to telegraph your moves, and hinders your balance. If you let your hips drive, it's easier to sink your weight, and you are less likely to over extend and lose your balance. It is also easier to feel rooted. Think of yourself as a driven screw: as you rotate, you sink into the ground and become ever more rooted. As we become rooted this way, we can use the ground as leverage to develop power for the strike.

HEAD

Keep your head up and your eyes level. Think of the crown of your head as suspended by a string from above. Keep your chin slightly tucked in. There are many reasons to keep your head upright. As we mentioned, there is the question of balance. If your head is over your shoulders and your shoulders are over your hips, it will be easier to lower your center of gravity and keep your balance.

Second, students who look down tend sometimes to lead with their head as though they were a bull or a ram trying to clash with their horns. They also have the tendency to move from their shoulders only instead of moving with the whole body. Your balance is easily lost or taken that way.

SHOULDERS

Allow your shoulders to roll forward ever so slightly. Seat your shoulders solidly in their sockets. You don't want to puff up the chest or raise the shoulders. At the very least, doing so affects you on a more physical level. Doing so disengages your shoulders from the rest of the body, tends to promote injury to your shoulders, and reduces your strike power. It also tends to disconnect moving from the hips. Raising your shoulders tends to encourage you to overreach your strike or overextend. It also tends to raise your breathing into the chest, which restricts your breathing and drains your energy. Instead, seat your shoulders firmly in their sockets. One way to find this is to stand with your elbows bent, palms up. Without flexing your chest, push your elbows down.

One other thing about the shoulders. Many of the old texts talk about keeping a space in your armpits. They suggest that you should think of it as keeping an egg in your armpits. Keeping that space allows your movements to be more expanded instead of collapsed. It tends to keep open the energy pathways between your shoulders and arms. Ideally, we don't want to crush the egg in your armpit, but you don't want to let it fall either.

EYES

Do not get caught up in the eyes of your opponent. Do not see your opponent's eyes or countenance. Do not see their physical size or muscles. Do not see their uniform or weapon, no matter how fearsome they might be. See only an obstacle in your way. See only your opponent's intent and center. Their core. See the disposition and distance of their hips and shoulders. Do not note whether your opponent is attractive or not. Regardless of how your opponent appears, see only an opponent. Size, muscle, and physical attributes of beauty are only impediments that will get in your way. They are noise and distraction. Strength and size may offer advantage, but by themselves, they do not overcome skill, training, or determination.

Sifu has said many times that there is no need to look at the sidewalk. You won't find your opponent there. And there won't be any instructions written in the concrete.

Others suggest that that you should keep your eyes directly on your opponent, that you need to be able to see what they are going to do. At the very least, keep your eyes on your opponent's center mass.

Sifu says never focus directly on your opponent's eyes. For one thing, if you are focused on their eyes, you will miss what they do with their hands, body or feet. You won't be listening. Sifu says that if you wait to see what your opponent is going to do before you react, it's too late. It takes too long. He is of the firm belief that if you move quietly and connect with your opponent, you can learn to tune into them. You can learn to read your opponent. He believes you should keep track of your opponent from the corner of your eye — through your peripheral vision.

Common wisdom suggests there is more to it than that. We know that snakes and cats use their eyes to sort of mesmerize their intended prey. Some people can do that too, beguile or enthrall people by catching and holding the gaze of their intended prey. We also know that a gaze can be inviting, intimidating, or creepy. According to folklore, the evil eye was supposed to be a curse you could project onto your enemies just with your eyes. Yes, the eyes can project emotions. More than that, animals and sensitive people can feel someone's gaze on them. There is most certainly an energy in the eyes. The eyes can project energy and receive it.

Science might want to weigh in on this discussion. It is commonly accepted that there are two kinds of vision: direct and peripheral. The two kinds of vision are very different. Direct vision distinguishes and interprets color and detail. Your direct vision connects directly to your thinking or rational mind, and it allows you to focus and read this most excellent Tai Chi book. Your eyes are taking the time to decipher the various shapes of the letters and decode the meanings of the words. Yes, your brain is doing a considerable amount of the work. It's worth noting that because direct vision is so connected to your rational thinking mind, the visual cortex, it does not inform you of everything in your environment. You become busy checking out the details but you may miss out on the big picture at the edges, the periphery of your sight.

Peripheral vision is very different. Peripheral vision doesn't decipher colors as well. It isn't meant to decipher details particularly well either. Instead, peripheral vision is adapted to detect movement at the edge of your focus and can operate in lower light conditions. Information taken in through the peripheral vision relates more to movement and distance than it does to details and colors. Use that to your advantage.

FEET

We don't really think or talk about the feet too often. They occupy real estate at the very far, distant end of the body away from the head, face, and eyes, which seem to get most of our attention. However, the feet can be super useful, particularly when it comes to understanding how we move. Consider the geography of the foot. There are six areas we want to think about. The first five relate to balance. Three are at the front of the foot: the pad of the big toe, the ball of the foot which is the knuckle of the big toe, and the knuckle of the fifth or pinkie toe. If you stand on your tip-toes, you may wobble a little bit between these points on the front of the foot. As your sense of balance improves, you can control which of these areas to put your weight on. Next, there is the thick fleshy ridge along the outside of the foot, and the heel. If you concentrate on the outside ridge of your foot, you can raise the arch of your foot. The heel is useful, as we have seen, for empty step.

The last point of the foot is the hollow in the middle of the foot. It's like the palm or cup of the hand. The cup of the foot typically has thinner skin and for many people is a ticklish point. However, like the hands, there is a strong energetic point in the cup of the foot. It is called the Bubbling Well, and according to Tai Chi wisdom, it is the point in the foot where energy is drawn up from the ground into the body.

Sifu says it is worthwhile to spend time thinking about the feet and playing with them. Rotate your weight and focus from one point to the next. Doing so may foster circulation in the feet and possibly ward off a host of foot-related infirmities.

BREATHING

Breathing is one of my favorite activities. I do it every day.

"To breathe is to live. To breathe fully is to live fully, to manifest the full range and power of our inborn potential for vitality in everything that we sense, feel, think, and do. Unfortunately, few of us breathe fully."[71]

Sifu says that worrying about the details breathing in Tai Chi should generally come later in the journey of understanding Tai Chi. Some teachers like to teach breathing techniques early. Sifu likes to teach breathing after other basics are mastered. His philosophy is pretty simple. For the beginning student, or for any student, the important thing to remember about breathing is simple: Do it. Breathe. Deeply and only as much as needed. For someone who is new to Tai Chi, there is already plenty to think about.

Don't worry too much at first about breathing — unless you find yourself not breathing at all or unless you are out of breath. Unconsciously holding your breath or not breathing deeply enough while you are trying to remember the next move in your form should be avoided. Just breathe.

A LITTLE MORE DETAIL ABOUT THE BREATH

With respect to Tai Chi and martial arts in general, use your breath to power your strikes. Exhale on strike or the extension move. Inhale on the relaxation or the contracting move or in preparation for the next strike. When you inhale strongly or sharply in preparation for a strike, you will want to keep your shoulders down and the rest of your chest at rest. You really do not want to get tagged by your

---

71   Lewis, The Tao of Natural Breathing for Health, Well-Being and Inner
        Growth, p. 17.

opponent while you are inhaling. Instead, breathe into your belly, not your chest. Having said that, it's still better to breathe and risk telegraphing than it is to hold your breath.

With respect to Qi Gong practice, breathing is the opposite. You aren't practicing a martial art. Here, the idea is generally to fill your lungs and so breathing is the reverse of what you would like to do in martial arts: Inhale on the expansion moves. The idea is that as you expand the body you create more space for your lungs to fill. For the contracting moves, the goal is to use the contraction in order to help us push all of the air out of the lungs. Having said all that, it's important to remember that this is a very simplified plan for breathing. While there are many esoteric breathing techniques, for now, let's keep it simple. Simple is good. It's a good place to begin.

For the student who is further along in their Tai Chi journey, if you no longer have to concentrate too hard to remember what to do next in your form, let me offer a few additional thoughts. We know that breathing supplies oxygen to the cells in the body on the inhale. And we know that the exhale carries away carbon dioxide and other wastes from the body. This is no big surprise. What you may not realize is that the breath is intimately connected to all of the systems of the body. Higher volume lung capacity and ease of airflow have been linked to greater vitality, greater heart function, greater cognitive function (what do you think about that?), better emotional health, and longer life in general.[72] Conversely, poor breathing habits have been shown to contribute to or worsen a broad range of health issues. The breath can regulate or dramatically alter your affective emotional state.[73] In other words, breathing can change what and how you feel in the moment. Breathing can help you return to a state of calm and emotional balance in the face of adversity. Attention to the breath can help with concentration. The issue is that many people don't give any thought or attention to their breathing.

---

72 Wayne and Fuerst, The Harvard Medical School Guide to Tai Chi, 2013, p. 166.

73 Kabat-Zinn, Jon. Full Catastrophe LIving: Using the Wisdom of Your Body and Mind to Face Stress, Pain, Illness. Bantam Books, 2013.

Let me offer a few thoughts about how breathing can affect the body. Here are five basic breathing patterns and their general affect on the state of being. Not all of them are desirable. Let me note that here, I have only offered a basic sketch.

1. A shorter inhale coupled with a calm, drawn-out exhale tends to have a calming affect.

2. A slow extended inhale coupled with a sharp exhale has the tendency to excite the nervous system and prepare the body for action.

3. Sipping your breath is a calm, shallow inhale and matching exhale, and it tends to calm the heart rate and blood pressure. It's a good pattern to use for quiet meditation or for when your doctor is about to take your blood pressure. At the same time, sipping your breath means you take in less oxygen. There may be moments during your day when this is not ideal.

4. Calm, deep breaths, rhythmic inhales and exhales, tend to energize the body, raise awareness of yourself and your environment, and focus the mind while remaining calm. This might be a good pattern for waking up or warming up. It might be a good pattern for shedding anxiety and improving your mental clarity. Remember: Most of the time, breathe into the belly instead of your chest.

5. Rapid, sharp, short inhales and exhales can build anxiety and lead to hyperventilation.

So how do we increase airflow and lung capacity? Draw full breaths into the belly then exhale fully. Belly breathing, or diaphragmatic breathing, pulls the diaphragm muscle down and creates space for the lungs to expand and draw in air.[74]

Current Western aesthetic paradigms of bodily health and beauty favor tight, flat, cut abdominal muscles. However, tight abs

---

74 Kabat Zinn, p. 47.

may be the result of over exercise or anxiety and may restrict the lungs' ability to expand to their full capacity. These same aesthetic paradigms encourage us to puff up the chest and raise the shoulders when we breathe deeply. Keep in mind that the rib cage and spine are relatively stiff and do not offer as much room to expand the lungs. Furthermore, as we get older, the ligaments that connect the ribs and spine and the bones themselves tend to become calcified, brittle, and stiff. This can further limit lung capacity if we breathe into the chest instead of the belly. One other thing to keep in mind is that in Tai Chi, we don't want to raise the shoulders. Instead, we want to move from a lower center of gravity. We want to move from the hips. Breathe into the belly.

Remember just a few paragraphs ago when I suggested that we keep the breathing pattern simple? Watch the breath and pay attention to what is going on in the body. Don't worry too much about controlling the breath unless you are specifically interested in calming yourself. Just watch and feel.

"Let the body breathe you."[75]

Models of the Body

Models are really useful tools for conceptualizing an abstract idea. In other words, models help us to better understand complex, complicated systems. The body itself is anything but an abstraction, but the interrelationship of all of the disparate pieces and parts of the body is more easily understood and much more available to understanding and self-inspection if we have one or more models to guide us. It's important to understand, though, that a model is really just a representation of an idea and not necessarily complete or comprehensive. Models may illustrate just one or two specific ideas.

With respect to Tai Chi, using models of the body can help us to better understand some of the core ideas. For example, why is it important to keep the head erect over the shoulders? And why is

---

75 Wayne and Fuerst, p. 171.

it important to keep the shoulders seated in their sockets and not tensed up alongside the ears? What happens in our body when we extend our arm?

I have three models for understanding how the body works. The first reflects paradigms common to Western medicine and Western ideas about how the body moves. It is mechanistic and reductionist in the sense that it focuses on the mechanism of various parts. However, I do not mean to suggest that the self or person is a mechanism in any way. The model simply refers to the way the body moves. The Clockwork Model is only meant to illustrate how to move the body to gain biomechanical advantage. The second model, the Fabric Model, embodies a more Eastern, more wholistic view of the body. This one is organismic. It considers the body as a complete organism. For the purpose of better understanding Tai Chi, I would also like to offer an idea about structure called the Four Points Theory. The Four Points Theory illustrates ideas about structure and balance.

I want to point out that these three ideas are very different from each other. Indeed, they may even contradict either other. There is nothing wrong with that. We don't want to think about all of them at the same time. Each one illustrates different ideas. Each of them have different things to teach us. When you read this, imagine for a moment what moving your body might be like if you followed one or the other of these models. How might thinking about one or the other affect the way you move? Is there a difference between them?

THE CLOCKWORK MODEL OF THE BODY

The Clockwork Model builds on our discussion of structure. However, it leads us to different ideas. It's the view of the body as a mechanical device like a clock. It illustrates the theory of biomechanical advantage, which means simply coordinating various body parts to generate the greatest amount of power, regardless of the availability of huge muscles. It can help you generate leverage, torque, rooting, balance, and so on.

Imagine the mechanism of a clock. It comprises interconnected gears, pulleys, weights, and rods. Our bodies are made up of a collection of interconnected of mechanical pieces: ball joints, articulated rods (limbs), cords (muscles), gears, and weight centers (the hips and feet). From this model, we can easily imagine all of the basic machines of levers, pulleys, gears, screws, and counterweights. All of these operate in conjunction to maximize our ability to move efficiently, gracefully, to remain balanced, or to apply power for a strike. The body can be viewed as mechanical if we think of it as being driven by pieces and parts.

Specifically, the idea is to use the feet for leverage against the ground (rooting) to generate power and torque through the feet, legs, hips, and core. We can use that, in turn, for various strikes and defensive moves, and they get expressed by the extension of the shoulders, elbows, hands or hips, knees, and feet. We can also use this theory to illustrate how to absorb a certain amount of incoming energy. We can use the body almost like a spring or shock absorber to absorb a certain amount of energy and transmit it to the ground. We can also use the spring or shock absorber idea to draw energy from the ground and transmit it through the arms and hands.

When it comes to healing or injury repair, all of these interconnected mechanical pieces and parts most often come to our attention when we feel any sort of dysfunction, dis-ease, dis-ability, pain, or stiffness. When we feel pain in our knees, shoulders, hips, or whatever, we tend to think that the problem is localized and related to that particular part. Western medical science favors the clockwork model because it is very good at identifying, repairing, or replacing various individual parts as problems with those parts arise.

How does this help in our discussion about Tai Chi? The point of Tai Chi is that we are learning to move with precision and intention. We are learning how to move more efficiently and at the same time, we are learning how to physically manipulate ourselves or, perhaps, an opponent. We are also learning about the physical structure of the body and how to use it to our advantage. We talked about the theory of structure, which is about remaining stable and maintaining functional balance while moving.

The Clockwork Model helps us, for example, to imagine keeping the head upright while we turn the hips. Think of the body as a screw. We "screw" ourselves into the ground to generate leverage with the feet. As the foot is pressed into the ground, it anchors the hips to rotate. The rotation of the hips is connected to the turn of a foot. The "gear" that runs the hips can also be connected to the joints of articulation in the arms. The arms, of course, can extended or rotated. We connect turning the hips with the leverage of the feet and the extension or expression of energy through the rods —the arms or legs. This is what we mean by the phrase that moves are anchored in the feet, driven by the hips, and expressed through the hands.

The Clockwork Model illustrates how to apply the concepts of the basic machinery of physics: leverage, distributed load, rotation, potential energy, and so on to the body to achieve biomechanical advantage. In other words, we want to make use of basic mechanical principles to maximize the power and efficiency of movement. As one wheel or gear turns, it connects to and turns, extends, or rotates other gears, screws, rods, or weights. In other words, all of the disparate parts of the body move in conjunction and with common effect in order to generate the most efficient work while expending the least possible amount of energy.

LET'S TALK ABOUT THE HAND, ELBOW, AND SHOULDER FOR A MOMENT.

There is quite a lot that can be said for the position of the hand with respect to its relationship to the elbow, shoulder, and body center. First, if your elbow is pointing down and closer to your body, then it is more likely, but not certain, that your shoulder will be properly seated in its socket. At the same time, you don't want your elbow to be pressed against your side. Remember, you want a sense of expansion. You want to avoid a sense of collapse of your arm against your body. As I pointed out earlier, many of the old texts talk about maintaining a space in your armpit, as though you are carrying an egg under your arm. Maintain that space. Don't crush the egg. Don't allow it to fall either. This sense allows you to maximize your biomechanical advantage and keep your energetic pathways from collapsing as well.

This is a more efficient posture for generating power in pushes or strikes and for absorbing impact from outstretched hands. A stronger connection between shoulder and body means you can more efficiently use the entire body to generate power or absorb impact. Of course, there are times when your elbow is raised and pointed out. Having the flexibility to raise your shoulder if you want to can be really useful as well.

If the hands are too close to the chest, it may come with a sense of collapse of your working space. That collapse often coincides with a decline in power generation. It represents disengaged leverage.

There is an equally dangerous if opposing trap of hyperextending or locking the elbow out. Hyperextension can injure the tendons or ligaments in the elbow or arm. Worse, impact against an hyperextended elbow can result in a broken elbow, damaged tendons, dislocated shoulder, or a wicked arm bar. Keeping a slight bend in the elbow can help to absorb the energy of impact if you should fail to transfer your energy properly. On the other hand, if you can manipulate your opponent into hyperextending their elbow, you can use it to your advantage. You could either break their elbow or manipulate their shoulder to distort their balance or structure.

The ideal position for generating efficient movement, therefore, is to have the elbow at the side of the body about a fist's distance away. Of course, we move the arm and the elbow in and out of that position. The ideal working distance for a hand strike, for example, is for the elbow to remain about a fist's distance from the body. Of course, this is a rule of thumb — more like a guideline than an actual rule. There are plenty of times when it is appropriate to move the elbow closer or further away. With respect to the clockwork model of the body, the greatest leverage and biomechanical advantage comes when we realize the connection between the elbow and the body center.

I point these out to illustrate the point. My explanation here is meant to be no more than a sketch. There is plenty more information available for you to explore. Your teacher will be able to help you explore this further.

Here is a more specific example: Chin Na is a subdiscipline of Tai Chi. It makes specific use of the clockwork model to understand how to employ and engage joint locks, bone manipulations, and throws. For example, suppose your opponent grabs your wrist tightly and won't let go. We can use the clockwork model to illustrate how to find the weak point in their grip and how to rotate our own wrist to exploit their weakness and escape. Essentially, we can apply our biomechanical advantage to their disadvantage. We know that the weakest point of their grip, no matter how strong they are, is the thumb. We can change the yaw of our wrist — the side-to-side movement — to apply counterpressure against the thumb and break their grip.

However, there is more. We can use the principles of biomechanical advantage—that is, the clockwork model — to understand how coordinating the feet, hips, shoulders, and elbow into one single move both increases our leverage against our opponent's grip and reduces the amount of strength we need to break free. And furthermore, executing this move with the proper intent can help us to escape their grip, then coil our body and generate potential energy — stored up energy, ready to be unleashed — for a follow-up strike if we choose.

THE FABRIC MODEL OF THE BODY

"If you want to make the claim that you want to be healthy, know where your parts are; know how you are woven together."[76]

---

76 My thanks to my friend Neil B. Anderson, LMT, and student of the internal arts, for sharing his vision of the fabric model of the body with me.

This second model presents the body as a fabric, or a woven web. Imagine the body as a tapestry of interwoven threads: nerves, blood vessels, organs, Qi energy meridians, and fascia. By the way, fascia is that fibrous material that sheathes all of the organs, bones, muscle bundles and nerves. If you pull on one part of the fabric, or pull a thread out of the weave, it will tug on a distant part of the body. Or if you press on the foot, for example, the foot, you can establish a sense of connection through out the body and use it to extend the finger tips. Or you might stretch the extend the finger so that the foot comes along with it. Either way, we can think of it as using the entire body to move one finger.

The spine still represents the central core from which all of the other organs radiate and are suspended. It also represents the core pathway through which nervous impulse conduction radiates throughout the entire body. As I mentioned, if you pull on a thread at one point in the body, you can affect a distant part. It goes through the spine.

So how does this model apply to our discussion about Tai Chi? The fabric model illustrates a different concept for moving. We can use it to illustrate that the body flows. It highlights the idea of moving in circles and curves instead of straight lines. It offers the idea that gently stretching and compacting the various parts of the body can promote energy flow and nervous impulse conduction throughout the body. It also highlights the idea of using the whole body in a sort of wave for each move. For example, if we push with one hand, we want to activate the other hand. We might also push our feet into the ground with a feeling of engaging a line or a string from the heel through the legs, hips, waist, core, chest, and through the arms. This is how we connected the entire body. Everything is either contracting, curving, or expanding in coordinated purpose.

The fabric model illustrates the ideas of flow and intention. In other words, as you move through a particular move, the whole body flows in synchronization. Take Brush Knee, for example. It is typically executed as a push with one hand, but it could also be an elbow strike, a shoulder strike, or even a hip strike. The entire body flows into the execution of the move. The strike is powered by the entire body moving in coordinated intention and synchronization. The reason why is because the entire body is moving through the move every bit as much as the hands are.

For doctors of Traditional Chinese Medicine, the effects of a tug or pull on an energetic charge or load at one point of the body may travel throughout the body and cause a reaction elsewhere. This is precisely the theory behind acupuncture or the energy meridian system. Acupuncture, for example, might use a very thin needle at a specific point to open or access Qi energy flow to promote health. The inhibition or constriction of blood or Qi energy flow may cause dis-ease or dys-function in discrete parts of the body or even in nonspecific parts elsewhere. Health and well-being are achieved through efficient, unfettered energy flow.

There is also a subdiscipline of Tai Chi that makes a study of identifying and exploiting specific points along the energy meridians to cause damage. The idea here is to target these points and attack them for the purpose of disrupting energy flow throughout the body. To continue our metaphor of the body as fabric, the idea is to find and impact important "threads" so that Qi energy conduction is disrupted and severe damage is caused. Let me note a few things here. First, this is a very advanced and perhaps dark area of combat and it is well beyond the scope of this book, my expertise, or my willingness to say much more. Yes, Tai Chi is, in part, a means to study of Qi energy conduction throughout the body. The knowledge contained in Tai Chi can be used either cause damage or to heal. However, there is a very long, disciplined journey ahead before you get to that point. If you short cut the journey and try to jump too far ahead, you run a serious risk of causing great harm. The better way of looking at it is to use Tai Chi to move through the world in harmony with ourself, others, and our environment.

THE FOUR POINTS THEORY

The Four Points Theory can shed some light on why all of this is important. The Four Points Theory is one way to conceptualize how structure and balance work within the body. And so, it illustrates the idea of structure and balance in greater detail.

Before we get into the Four Points Theory, let's make a quick sketch at how the body is configured. Looking at the skeleton, the top down, we begin with our heavy, bulbous skull. Obviously, the skull houses and protects a three-and-a-half-pound mass called the brain. The skull rests at the top of a long stem, the spine. Briefly stated, the spine sprouts from the base of the skull. As we mentioned, all of the disparate parts of the body radiate and are suspended from the spine. The shoulder girdle is suspended from the spine just below the neck. The arms hang from the shoulders. The shoulder girdle also includes the clavicle (collarbone), the shoulder joints, the scapulae (shoulder blades), and so on. The clavicle connects to the sternum, which helps to support the rib cage from the front. The ribs also sprout from the spine in back. Lower down, the spine connects with the hip girdle. The coccyx or tail bone is the end of the spinal column. Nevertheless, hips are not only the juncture of the bones that become the legs, but they are also sort of the juncture box for all of the blood vessels, nerves, tendons, ligaments, and so on. These wind their way through the hips and extend down into the legs.

Each of the models features the spine as the central construct, around which all of the disparate parts rotate, radiate, or are suspended. Your range of motion is determined by the limits of your skeleton, your flexibility (which is largely represented by the fascia), and by the limits of stretching and compressing tissues and organs.

The Four Points Theory begins with recognition of the spine as the flexible, central core of the body around which everything rotates. It is based on the simple idea that the distortion or distention of the spine can result in loss of structure, balance, and one's ability to move or launch a strike. The four points in question are each of the shoulders and hips. Specifically, two are at the junction of the chest and the two shoulders. There is a sort of crease there between the shoulders and the chest. The other two are the junctures between the torso and the two sides of the hips. The chin or head plays a role, as well, in the sense that it can be used to distort the shoulders. As we have seen, every move in Tai Chi is rooted in the feet, controlled by the hips and expressed through the hands. From a physiological point of view, the four points maintain the balance and structure of the whole body. If any of these points are distorted, disrupted, or moved out of place, then the structure and balance of the entire body is affected and may collapse. The more points that are distorted, the more severely the whole body may be thrown off balance. While it is certainly possible to break someone's structure by distorting one point, distorting two points is clearly more effective.

For this reason, it is enough to suggest that most of the time, as I mentioned, we want to keep the head over the shoulders, the shoulders over the hips. These are elements of good structure. Humor me for a moment and read those last couple of sentences again: Most of the time, we want to keep the head over the shoulders and the shoulders over the hips. Most of the time.

Of course, there are exceptions. Some kicks, for example, require us to counterbalance the extending leg by leaning slightly. Stepping out behind or to the side of our body and putting the heel down first may require a slight lean as well. However, even in those cases, we want to keep the hips grounded. We want to have the hips be a sort of ballast pushing down through the legs and feet. We have talked about rooting. Even if you lean over a bit, you can still be rooted. Think of it as the ballast that keeps a ship upright in heavy seas.

There are guidelines for the knees as well. When you are standing, your knees should bend in the direction that your toes are pointing and the knees should not extend past the toes. Otherwise, you may put too much pressure on the knees and injure them. Furthermore, in Tai Chi, when we turn the foot, we most often do so by lifting the toes and rotating on the heel. Rarely, we might lift the heel and rotate on the ball of the foot. However, either way, be intentional and mindful about this. Otherwise, the sole of your shoe might catch on the carpet or floor, and you could easily twist and injure your knee.

As we've discussed, we want to rotate the hips and shoulders as we move. We want to coordinate all of the parts of the body to move in unified, common purpose — even if the various parts are moving at different speeds. However, we want to be certain that as we twist, we keep the body upright as though we are a screw that is being driven upright into a piece of wood. The shoulders, for example, shouldn't dip, distort, extend, or raise up by the ears as we move. It's important to think of the shoulders and hips rotating around the spine.

The Four Points Theory becomes particularly important with respect to conflicts in which grappling, throws, joint locks, or manipulations come into play. Part of the genius of Tai Chi is that it offers answers to all of those strategies. In the branch of Tai Chi called Chin Na, the idea is to respond by listening to the intent of your opponent and moving ahead of them into the manipulation of the body—commonly hips, shoulders, wrists, elbows or knees. However, the other thing to keep in mind is that when you are off balance, get your hips beneath you.

There is a more ordinary application for the Four Points Theory, as well that will help in cases where you might otherwise lose your balance. Maybe you trip over something. Maybe you put your foot down on an uneven surface and roll your ankle. Maybe you slip. In these cases, yes, there may be injury to toe or ankle, but the greater problem is that you may have distorted your hips, lost your structure, and potentially created a more serious fall. Avoid this by learning to drop your hips under you as you fall and keep them under you as much as possible and drop down onto your knees. Of course, all of this relates to balance.

A Mystery for Your Consideration

So why is posture, structure, and all of this important? Well, allow me to present a mystery for your consideration. Traditional Chinese Medicine has been confidently and successfully studying the Qi energy meridians, pathways, and reservoirs for some five thousand years. They have based their medical understanding and treatment of disorders on this paradigm. They have been very successful at it. Indeed, they have very accurate physical depictions of Qi energy pathways and the attending acupuncture points along those pathways used to manipulate the body's energy flow.

Add to this two additional points of information. First, Western medical science can easily present extraordinarily detailed representations of nerves and blood vessels. It can detect and identify an electro-energetic field that permeates and surrounds the body. It is also well aware that various organs — most notably the heart and the brain, but others, too—generate their own electro-energetic field. However, Western medical science cannot seem to find any physical evidence for this system of energy pathways — meridians — and their attendant reservoirs.

Traditional Chinese Medicine, on the other hand, has a very detailed understanding of meridians. However, they have, at best, a very rudimentary representation of the complex and indeed rather obvious (to us) system of blood vessels and nerves.[77] Doesn't that sound odd? Why doesn't Traditional Chinese Medicine have a detailed understanding of blood vessels, for example? How do we reconcile these different understandings? Perhaps this is a case in which a system becomes so embroiled in its own idiomatic expression that it misses information that is not contained in its vocabulary. In other words, maybe Western medical science is so preconditioned to identify various physical pieces and parts that it misses the spaces in between. Maybe they miss the interrelationship, the interactivity of the different pieces and parts. The traditional Chinese system uses

---

77 Kaptchuck, The Web That Has No Weaver

different metaphors and idioms to understand the functioning of the body. Keep in mind that medicine is not my expertise. We are wandering just a little into conjecture here.

And there is more. My hypothesis is that the different materials that make up the fabric of the body present varying levels of electrical or energetic resistance, conduction, and storage. Maybe Qi energy flows easily along conductive tissues and is slowed and therefore shaped by tissues that are more electric-impulse resistant. My guess is that fascia is more energy resistant. These fibers aren't served by nerves the way muscle bundles and organs are. They also appear to have natural energy resistance because they sheath everything, contain everything. Nerves, of course, are more energy conductive. However, the signals they transmit are specialized and not perhaps related to Qi.

Think of it this way. If we want to bring water to a house, we can create a system of pipes and make water flow through it. On the other hand, if you've ever seen a weepy, seepy, damp basement, you'll know that water doesn't really need pipes to find pathways through cinderblocks and baseboards. Instead, it draws and puddles in low areas and flows along water conductive pathways. We typically refer to these pathways as cracks in the foundation. You won't find them on architectural plans of the house. And if you have cracks and leaks in the walls of your basement, you would not call a plumber because they would want to look for pipes — not cracks. How much sense does that make?

At the same time, for the energy to flow through your body, you have to pay attention to your posture, structure, and balance. With respect to Qi flow throughout the body, we have to open the channels — widen the cracks, so to speak — so it can flow. Simply put, the leaky basement metaphor represents good Qi flow, health, and well-being.

One last note on this for now. The discussion about Chin Na or Qi energy manipulation that I have presented here is meant for illustrative purposes only and not for instruction in method. If you are interested in learning about them, my recommendation is to have a conversation with your teacher.

Chapter 11: **Mind**

Class this morning was horrible. I moved through my forms like a tree stump. My limbs were made of wood. It might have been the result of a late night or the creaks of cold, tight muscles. My Tai Chi was stiff and brittle. Often, when my body feels this way, my mind gets stuck in darkness and doubts. My emotions and my thinking are every bit as stiff and brittle as my body. In times like these, it is tempting to linger in the shadows and think dark thoughts rather than seek the sunlight. It kind of feels disgusting, particularly in the morning. I have come to believe there is a correlation: When the body is stiff, the mind is foggy, at best. The mind mirrors the body. And unless I change it, it can affect the entire day. So...I change it.

Look. The greatest tool we possess to create change — positive or negative — to adapt to a changing environment, to survive, and to thrive is this three-pound-ish gelatinous mass that we carry between our ears. The brain is considered by contemporary Western paradigms to be the physical representation of the mind, though other traditions that are more wholistic include the heart, as well. Nevertheless, we can use our minds to improvise tools, create new ways of doing things, and even change the way we see the world. We can change the rules of engagement to our advantage. Our mind can also allow ego, fear, anger, and darkness control us. The human mind is capable of achieving great things, and it is capable of great destruction. How can we use it to answer questions like these? And what does this have to do with Tai Chi?

If you are thinking about doing Tai Chi, are you doing Tai Chi? If you fear getting hit, you are not doing Tai Chi. If you fear getting hit, it is likely you will get hit. If you fight, you will probably get hit regardless. So why worry about it? If you become consumed by fear of falling, well, guess what will happen next. Embrace your fear. Face it. Replace it with intention. It is only noise. You cannot listen if all you hear is noise.

Of course, we all have moments of distraction. We all have moments when thoughts and doubts sneak in. We're checking out that pretty person over there. (Are they impressed?) Our teacher is watching us move through the form; he's got his critical eyebrow raised. Suddenly, we stumble over Brush Knee or some other move. It happens to everyone. It happens to me all the time. In one sense, it's a good thing that it does. These moments can teach us valuable things. They remind us that if we become distracted during our moves, we have more training to do. They remind us of our humanity and humility. We are not perfect beings. If we were, we wouldn't be any fun. They teach us to feel and be aware without being consumed by emotions. These moments teach us the difference between the Void and the Abyss.

Here's a key point, however. Yes, these moments have something to teach us. We experience them. Then how quickly can we return our concentration to the task at hand?

Concentration

One of the early lessons of Tai Chi concerns how to better concentrate, how to focus our attention on a given activity. That concentration might be focused with laser-like precision on one particular idea or intention. It might be diffuse and aware of the environment in general. With respect to Tai Chi, we need to acquire the understanding the body comes first. Then, we can acquire understanding of the mind. Understanding the spirit comes later still. Move slowly through your form. Then, move slower, yet. This will develop your concentration skills. Of course, slowing down is more difficult. It takes ever more concentration, greater focus, greater guard against monkey mind (coming up). You are not only slowing down your movement, you are also learning to affect the focus and concentration of your mind.

There are many things you can choose to focus your mind on while you are moving through your form. You might begin with concentrating on which move comes next. If that is the case, then perhaps you don't know your form as well as you might like. Which is fine. It takes practice. You might choose to engage with imaginary opponents while you move through your form. In that case, every move represents a defense or attack application. Every move has its established or commonly recognized applications. Other possible applications are hidden. They are more difficult to find. I like to look for creative or alternative applications as I move through my form. Another option is to concentrate on sensing the people and the room around you. This might begin as an exercise of the imagination. As you move through the form, can you find, feel, or sense, the people in class with you? If you are practicing at home, can you find your cat as you move through the form? Yet another option is to concentrate on the energy, the Qi, within you as you move through your form. Of course, you don't have to follow the same one every time. Having said that, some of these are fairly sophisticated or advanced options. For one thing, they require you to know your form well enough so that you don't have to think about what move comes next.

Here is the next question: What is going on in your head while you are practicing Tai Chi? What you choose to think about, focus on, or concentrate on while you practice your form colors the impact that your practice will have on developing or changing your neural pathways. Speaking more plainly, how you choose to occupy your mind while you practice will color your mental and emotional habits throughout your entire day and all the days beyond. When you practice, will you choose balance? Calmness? Compassion? Grace? Gratitude? Anger?

The Avatars of Emotion

It's an old story. An old Cherokee man was teaching his grandson, and he said to the boy this: "Listen. Two wolves are at war within my heart. One is bright, wise, kind, and patient. He is the wolf of abundance and love. The other is dark, jealous, angry, and selfish. He is the wolf of scarcity and fear."

The boy asked his grandfather, "Grandfather, which one will win?"

Grandfather replied, "Which one will win is the one that I feed."

The mind is a noisy place. The wolves are always barking and growling at each other. Listening to them can be painful and noisy. It can reveal unpleasant truths.

Take a moment, though. Feel each of those wolves. Feel their strength and their power within you. Which one is stronger? Which one would you like to feed today? You can learn to master your attention. Or you could allow social media, television, the cell phone, sources of external noise to drown out the voices of the wolves in your heart. You could allow these things to master your attention. In fact, in our consumer-driven society, it seems there are endless voices clamoring for our attention, all the time. This noise will gladly move in and make a home in your head if you allow it. What if you don't want to allow that?

Habits of Mental Behavior

Allow me to offer a model of mental health. We talked about models a moment ago. A model is really only a construct, a representation that facilitates discussion and conceptualization. It offers a vocabulary that allows us to discuss problems and challenges. Earlier, we talked about models for thinking about the body. Now, this particular model relates to mental health and is perhaps overly simplistic. Nevertheless, I offer it for the purpose of helping us to better understand Tai Chi. It is simply this: The state of our mental health comprises our collected habits of mental and emotional behavior.

Of course, this model sets aside mental and emotional needs like self-understanding, connection, community, diet, exercise, biochemistry, and story. On the other hand, I mean to say that we often find ourselves responding to and interpreting situations and experiences in a repetitive manner that becomes familiar, indeed habitual, whether effective or not, useful or not. I also mean to suggest that habits, as difficult as they are to change, are indeed changeable.

For example, how do you typically respond when someone tells you "no?" What thoughts and emotions do you experience? Do you feel rejected? Dejected? Frustrated? Angry? Maybe these are responses that have become habituated. You turn to them even before you have all of the information. Likely, you don't really know why you were told no. Maybe it has nothing to do with you. Maybe the person is telling you no because they are looking at something else that is very important to them. Maybe they are looking at something you don't see. Maybe they don't have enough information about what you are asking. What if you draw your conclusions based on preconceived notions about yourself or your world—your mental habits. Suddenly, emotions and self preconceptions have clouded your judgement. What if you could change your habitual response and look at things differently?

But there is another way of looking at noise in your mind. The mind is constantly active. The neurons in the brain are always firing — even if we aren't always aware of it. As they do, habits of thinking become entrained. The more focus and attention that we give to particular thoughts, the louder they seem to become. And of course, the louder thoughts are the ones that draw our attention more. The loudest "voices" of neurons firing in our brain begin to crowd out everything else. Which wolf will you feed?

This is part of the reason that habitual thoughts and strong emotions always seem to take over: love, anger, fear, sadness, lust, joy. And when they do, we often use words to describe them like addictive, intrusive, obsessive, overwhelming, or all-consuming. In other words, these emotions can completely crowd out other thoughts and ideas—as though covering us in a wet woolen blanket of experience.

Learn to recognize the noise or this: Often, when we talk about emotions, we say "I am angry" or "I am happy" as though we, ourselves, embody these emotions. Imagine standing at the top of a cliff shaking your fists at the heavens — "I am angry!" — as if anger is some petty god who momentarily steals every bit of personality and individuality you posses. And it does. Sometimes, raging at the Cosmos feels good. Sometimes, it is useful. Sometimes, we really need to do it. If that's your situation, do it. Let it out. Then put it away. Unchecked anger possesses you. You become "Angry." You become the Avatar of Anger. And all the world shall tremble. You are no longer you.

Or we "fall in love" as though "Love" is a cliff that we somehow wander off. And of course, anyone who has ever been in love would say that the dizzying emotions seem very much like falling from a great height. To be sure, love is a beautiful madness. And people do it every day. You get the point.

To be clear, I am not suggesting that we deny ourselves the experiences of anger, fear, or love. Not at all. Recognizing our emotions is a healthy response to our experience. Experiencing emotions is one of the greatest gifts of being alive. If we didn't experience our emotions, the world would be a bland, boring place. Just don't let your emotions eat you.

ONE MORE TIME: DON'T LET YOUR EMOTIONS EAT YOU

The truth is, you cannot "do" Tai Chi if you are consumed by depression, anger or anxiety. You just can't. It's OK. Calm yourself. If you are angry and you try to practice Tai Chi, the art will tell you. If you are depressed or anxious, it will tell you. It has a way of revealing these things. At the same time, if you are feeling angry, depressed, or anxious, then do your Tai Chi anyway. Begin with a single step if you like. You may be in for a happy surprise.

Instead, how much different would our experience of emotions be if we spoke of them without self-identification but only identification of the feeling: "I feel angry" or "I'm experiencing happiness?" Simply by expressing your emotional state in similar terms to having an experience means that you hold onto the core center of yourself while you are enjoying these experiences.

Something else to consider is this. What would it be like to walk into an argument with a mindset of focus, connection, and curiosity? How would that be different from walking into an argument with rage, anger, fear, or dread? What if you were confident that you could answer any conflict or challenge? How would that be different? At least if we recognize fear and let it go, we won't also have to fight that dark, angry wolf nipping at our heels. How do we manage our fear? How do we change our mindset?

This is part of the reason why internal arts like meditation and Tai Chi are so important. They teach us to separate the noise and listen to the still, small voice within. They teach us to regain our connection to beings around us, even if — especially if — they intend us harm.

Know Your Opponent, but Do Not Let Them Know You

Consider another dimension of mind. Tai Chi wants to teach you awareness of subtle things. There are many things that we can only sense or feel. That doesn't mean we are necessarily conscious of them or aware of them, or even that we pay attention to them. Feelings represent sensory inputs: messages received in response to various stimuli. We get messages about our internal thoughts and experiences. Feelings might also be messages about external or environmental experiences and perceptions. We might have feelings about something that someone said. Feelings might be the energy of anticipation of an experience. Feelings might include awareness of your state of being or awareness of others around you.

Then we give name to our feelings and something odd happens. We give name to our feelings and they become emotions. The anticipation of an oncoming experience, for example, could be excitement or anxiety. Which name we choose to give it colors the way we think about the experience, how we perceive it, and how we respond to it. Excitement and anxiety, of course, are very similar. In the face of challenge, we can feel excitement or we can feel anxious and wish to avoid it.

Most often, we name our feelings before we are even aware of them. Instantaneously. Most often, the names we give to our feelings are habitual. If we are used to naming a feeling a certain way, it becomes a well-worn path and an easier one to follow. The more we talk about or allow ourselves to sink into "our anxiety," for example, the stronger the habituated mental pathway becomes. The wolf we usually feed, learns to eat first.

On the other hand, with awareness and determination, we can replace instinctual emotional choices with those of our choosing which are more advantageous. We can choose to feed whichever wolf we want.

Emotions take on an energetic aspect which are radiated, expressed, or repressed. Emotional energy can be "heard" or felt by sensitive others. We can feel the emotions that others radiate. We can even influence others by the emotions that we radiate. Strong emotions such as rage or love can raise the ambient emotional energy between people. Projecting or emoting calmness, patience, or gratitude can lower it. Calmness, patience, and gratitude can even open the door to alternative or creative responses to challenge. Repressed energy or energy hidden in the body can become trapped in the body and affect health and wellbeing.

Ultimately, we want to increase our sensitivity to feelings and become aware of our emotions and those of others. This is what we mean by the phrase "know your opponent, but don't let him know you." Feel your opponent's emotions, but choose yours. This is the science of self-awareness.

First of two monkeys: Monkey Mind

In my head sometimes lives a crazy little monkey. He bounces around, scrabbles for tasty morsels to chew on, and chitters for attention. Monkey mind is a term used in meditation that describes moments when our concentration is interrupted by unassociated impulses: thoughts, feelings, cravings, or other distractions. The monkey most often appears during moments of meditation, when we are trying hard to relax our mind or focus our attention. Relax harder. It has been said that you cannot stop the brain from thinking. Nor would you want to. Neurons in the brain fire constantly. Some of these impulses control autonomic functions. They regulate systems that we don't really think about such as heart rate, breathing, digestion, and so on. We can set those aside for the moment.

We are still subject to intrusive brain impulses. When we relax the mind, quiet impulses are released to bubble to the surface. Feelings. These may include intuitions of various kinds, creative or cognitive insights, or distractions. The idea is to sift through these impulses and separate what is useful from what is distracting. Ironically, when we struggle to push the distracting thoughts away, when we try hard to ignore them, they usually become louder and more disruptive. Distractions are like that small monkey. If they think you aren't listening to them, they get louder and more insistent. They drown out intuitions, creative impulses, focus, and the quiet serenity of a calm mind. If struggling to subdue the monkey makes him louder and more insistent, how do we control him? How do we return to the meditative state?

We can't beat the monkey into submission. Yelling at him, pushing him away just makes him louder and more insistent. Instead, we have to acknowledge him. We must listen to him, pet him, and cuddle him until he quietly settles onto our lap. Acknowledge your distractions and let them go in peace.

With respect to Tai Chi, and perhaps higher levels of mediation, taming the monkey mind means organizing and prioritizing our cognitive functioning. At its highest levels, it isn't about weeding out ruminations, distractions, intrusive thoughts, and emotions. It is about figuring out what is noise. It's about listening to that still, small voice—the voice of intuition and understanding. We want to catch our intuitions and insights. The aim is to recognize them, to separate them from the noise, and give voice to them.

With respect to Tai Chi, we are aiming to connect with our opponent, feel them, understand their intentions before they do. The point of conquering the monkey mind is to learn how to listen to each thought, each feeling, each fleeting flash of cognitive motion and to attend to the ones that are useful while gently dismissing or dissolving the ones that are not.

Remember early in this book, I mentioned a few riddles and paradoxes? There is a classic Tai Chi paradox that says, in conflict, know your opponent, but do not let them know you. I think it means this: See your opponent's monkey mind. See their distractions, emotions, uncertainty, and confusion. If you listen, they might reveal these to you. You may choose to exploit them or you may choose to help your opponent find balance. Either way, don't let your opponent see your monkey. The point is not to squash or squelch your doubts and fears. The point is to find calm and balance despite your doubts and fears. Accept them. Embrace them. They are part of you. Then allow them to float away.

Second Monkey: Besotted Monkey Tai Chi

Listen. In the days before I began my first hundred-day challenge, there was a woman I wished to impress. She was everything that the object of one's unrequited affections usually is. She was dreamy: beautiful, intelligent, kind, modest, and so on. I'm pretty sure that all of the forest creatures happily helped her clean her cottage. This woman was the whole package. She only had one flaw in her personality, and it was a total deal-breaker: She had horrible taste in men. By that, I mean she had no interest in me. Simply put, her eyes were elsewhere.

Back then, I was a beginning practitioner of Tai Chi. I only had a few years of study under my belt. That woman? She might have watched me practice one time. She loved to dance. She was naturally graceful. She intuitively understood movement and body mechanics. I have no idea what she might have thought as she watched me practice. She might have politely said, "Wow, that was really good" and silently thought something else. And though I might not have wanted to admit it, at the time, I had a beginner's mind, a beginner's sense of skill, and movement. Worse, I was also trying to capture her attention and impress her. Which means that I probably moved through my form like a besotted monkey with one wooden foot and one foot in a roller skate. I'm sure you know what I mean. And that is precisely the point.

The reality of it is this: When you are doing Tai Chi and thinking about impressing a woman (or anyone, for that matter), are you really doing Tai Chi? No. You are feeding an emotion and that emotion is hijacking your attention. Not Tai Chi. In the case of trying to impress that woman, I was feeding my affection for her and my need for her attention, admiration, and approval. Emotions. Noise. So, of course, I probably looked like a besotted monkey. Not to worry though, I can laugh about it now. And note: We never want to ignore or repress our emotions. Emotions represent the gift of being human. Even unrequited affection can be a beautiful thing. Just don't let your emotions eat you.

Anyway, that's Tai Chi. It requires focus and being present. If you are feeding emotions while you are practicing Tai Chi, are you really "doing" Tai Chi? It's many, many hundreds of days later, and I have better understanding now than I did back then. Perhaps I even move better. When it comes to my daily practice, however, I no longer look around to see who is watching. That woman? Who knows where she ran off to.

The Switch

In class today, Sifu had each of us respond to a strike without much instruction. In turn, he threw a punch at each one of us to see how we would respond. Then, he told each of us to respond in Tai Chi form. For most of us, the difference between the two rounds of the exercise was profound. In the first round, we were pretty good at blocking, dissolving, or getting out of the way. In the second round, after being reminded to use our Tai Chi form, we moved quietly and calmly, with well-executed empty step. So the question is this: Why did we have to be reminded to use skills that clearly we possess?

In our discussion afterward, we talked about a Tai Chi switch. There is a cognitive function that needed to be performed first. Something had to be turned on before we could access the skill set we already have. Why is that? How do we learn to flip that switch in an instant so that the response of our choosing is habituated and instantaneous? So that those skills are available at a moment's need? Or is that even a thing? It's not only about conflict or challenge. Wouldn't it be better to move through the day and through the world with a sense of having the switch already turned on? In other words, wouldn't it be better to move through the day and the world with a sense of calm, balance, and readiness? How do we do that? That was, of course, the question of the day. Intention.

Here is a thought. Many people, me included, move through our day focused on a sense of self that represents the ego. The ego represents all of the objects of our identity that we are either born with or collect on our journey through life. These include the ways we think of ourselves, our view of our importance and esteem. It also includes all of our values. The ego is the part of the self that becomes wounded when we are insulted or slighted. It represents the construct of ourself that we must both defend and assert.

Ironically, when it comes to defense of the self, this part of us is exactly the part that we must turn off or disengage. It just is not useful for the defense of ourself. No only that, but it gets in the way of self-defense. So, when we are in class and Sifu challenges us, we want to answer in a way that impresses him. When it comes to impressing someone else, it is the ego and the emotions that we are appealing to and that is what causes us to move like a besotted monkey. What we are required to do is turn off the ego and engage the unthinking self.

Intention

It is often said that the journey of a thousand miles begins with a single step. I don't really believe that. The journey of a thousand miles begins with intention. If you don't begin with intention, you won't get very far. In other words, it's usually a good idea when planning your journey to ask yourself one simple question: Where do you want to go? If you don't know where you are going, don't be surprised if you don't get beyond your front yard. With respect to Tai Chi, however, you won't really know the destination of your journey because there is none. You may intend to learn Tai Chi, but the farther down that road you go, the more you realize that the light at the end is farther and farther away. That's ironic

You may ask yourself, what is my preferred response to this challenge? How do I avoid being eaten by my emotions? How do I change my mental habits? How do I flip the switch? These may be easy questions to ask, but they are not so easy to answer even if they seem so simple. Begin with intention. Begin with the idea that you intend to change your habits. Think about that. You need to know what you want to replace your current habits with. Fix that firmly in your mind. What do you want to be? What do you want to happen next? Fix your intention. Then, you also need to develop self-awareness in the moment. When you find yourself moving down the old path of flight, fight, or freeze, you need a course correction. You also need a mechanism for making that substitution. And then, you need to repeat until the new habit becomes…well, habit.

Tai Chi can help you develop awareness. It can offer the mechanism for change. Tai Chi wants to teach you new ways to move, so why not let it teach you new ways to be? Daily Tai Chi practice can offer the mechanism for repetition, the possibility to create new habits. This is why we are having this conversation. What you intend to become is your own decision to figure out.

The practice of Tai Chi — the thing you do at home — wants to teach you how to be aware. It will lead you to examine your mental and emotional habits. And your physical habits, too, such as how you move. As we mentioned, once you understand your form well enough to move through it without thinking about which move comes next, you can begin to turn your attention to other things. Tai Chi will reveal when your movement is inefficient. It will also reveal when your thoughts and emotions are intrusive. If, for example, you find yourself off balance and wobbly in a particular move, ask yourself why. What do you need to do to adjust it? What do you need to do find your balance? Maybe there is something on your mind that is causing a disturbance. Maybe you have unsettled feelings. Maybe your physical posture needs to be adjusted somehow. Ask yourself one simple question: Why are you off balance? Then listen for the answer.

Tai Chi also helps you cultivate the strength of your mind. First the discipline of daily practice builds will and intention. Certainly there are plenty of days when we don't feel like practicing, when distractions seem more appealing. Do it anyway. Build the will to master yourself despite whatever challenges you may face and master yourself. Then go out and master your world.

Ritual

Most often, we think of ritual as a spiritual practice. However, I am going to take a more cognitive approach and keep this discussion here within the section on the mind. Let's define ritual as an intentional activity that we use to build habits or to change our mindset or outlook. We use rituals to help us prepare for and improve prayer, practice, or performance. Different people might have a ritual before game play, before a recital, before writing, or even before bed. It's a systematized activity or collection of activities intended to adjust or affect your mindset. For example, a football coach might give a pregame pep talk in the locker room before the game starts. A writer might have a prayer or meditation ritual or some other task that helps them begin their writing practice. One of my Tai Chi mentors compares her daily practice to an "offering or prayer to the universe." It's a beautiful sentiment and a very spiritual point of view.

In my own practice, before I begin a form, I have my own ritual. I like to spend a moment finding and connecting with all of my various parts. I like to take a breath, set my intention, and repeat to myself the name of the particular form I am about to begin. Mine is a very body-mind oriented ritual. I wonder what other intentions I might set?

Other folks have a ritual of finding their feeling of Wuji before practicing their form. Repeated often enough, the ritual becomes a habit. It can change your mind. It becomes a powerful thing. What kind of mindset would you like to have for your Tai Chi practice? What kind ritual do you think might get you there?

Chapter 12: Qi

You may have heard of Qi. We talked about it just a moment ago with respect to the body. Here is a little more detail about this mysterious energy. Qi sounds quite a bit like chi in Tai Chi. Those words may sound alike, however, they are not related. The chi in Tai Chi refers to the "Grand Ultimate." On the other hand, Qi energy is analogous to life energy. It is the force or fuel that drives our bodily engines. The prevailing guideline is that you cannot cultivate or manipulate Qi energy circulation until you learn to become aware of it. Meditation, Tai Chi, and Qi Gong are the primary paths to awareness. I do think that other forms of exercise, nutrition, proper sleep, and other healthy habits can help us build Qi. At their core, both Tai Chi and Qi Gong represent the study and development of Qi.[78]

According to Chinese historical accounts, the study of Qi energy began some four thousand years ago. Not long after that, the cultivation of Qi was recognized as an element of health and well-being. Later still, Chinese thinkers began to study Qi as an energy for powering strikes and defensive strategies. Simply put, Qi is energy. The ancient Chinese ideograph for Qi is a combination of the ideograms for rice and air or steam. That is, Qi energy is fueled by food. And like the Sanskrit word prana or the Hebrew word ruach, there is an aspect of Qi that refers to air.

---

78 Qi is pronounced chee. It's also important to note here, that Qi or Chi energy is not the same Chinese word or ideogram as found in Tai Chi or Tai Chi Ch'uan. Chi energy is, however, the same ideogram as in Qi Gong or Chi Kung. Chi energy can also appear in English as "Qi" or "Ki" and refers to internal energy which is the foundation of many traditional Asian martial arts.

The primary categories of Qi include heavenly Qi, earthly Qi, and human Qi. Heavenly Qi is the energy of the Cosmos. We might compare it to the radiation from the sun or from deep space. Earthly Qi is the energy we get from healthy food, from nature, the ground, and from all living things. We might compare this to the energetic feeling of being in an old growth forest, in the mountains, or standing by the sea shore watching the waves.

Variations of Qi might be compared to cosmic or solar energy or the its reflection from the moon or other planets. In fact, we might suppose that every celestial body reflects light and energy. This is Qi. The interplay of Heavenly and Earthly Qi is the message of the Yin Yang symbol, also called the Taiji. The third primary category of Qi is human Qi. Human Qi obviously sits in between heaven and earth. So from a cosmic perspective, Qi energy is said to fill the universe. Closer to home, it represents the energy of the earth. Closer still, Qi is the energy that animates the body and gives vitality to the self. More broadly speaking, as a form of energy, the idea of Qi has been paired with a variety descriptors and adjectives and can refer to almost any variety of energy: electrical, heat, wind, radiation, steam, and similar.

On a more prosaic level, a person's Qi plays a role in how they physically present. A person might have, for many reasons, a powerful or energetic presence. For example, we might describe someone as bright-eyed and bushy-tailed. They have a lot of Qi. Or they might seem moody, wilted, or worn-out. They lack strong Qi.

We hear stories, sometimes, in which masters of Qi energy can perform unusual feats. Some are said to use Qi energy to break concrete bricks on their heads or bend metal bars or spark a fire. I cannot say with any certainty whether those accounts are true. However, I can tell you that Qi energy is a foundational concept in traditional Chinese constructs of healing. It is used to heal both the self and others.

According to Traditional Chinese Medicine, Qi energy circulates through the body by a system of pathways or meridians and is stored in a series of reservoirs. There are 12 main meridians (and many lesser ones) and three primary reservoirs. Think of the meridians as a network of conduits through which energy is transmitted and via which various parts of the body are connected. A toe, for example, might be connected by one of these pathways to an organ, the liver perhaps. A pain in the toe might reveal clues about the health and functioning of the liver, so practitioners believe.

The most well known of the reservoirs is called the triple burner. These are three reservoirs, or Dan Tiens. The first, and most well known, is located a few finger widths below the navel and a couple of inches behind it. The second reservoir is located within the chest, about the solar plexus. The third is located behind the forehead, about the level of the brow between the eyes. In the West, we are familiar with these. We might feel a hot, roiling sense in the gut or a heaviness in the chest or an ache in our forehead. These may be related to feelings, responses to our experience, or they may be related to something altogether different. These are also analogous to three of the Chakras in the East Indian yoga system.

Traditional Chinese Medicine has been interested in meridians and reservoirs since it recognized Qi thousands of years ago.[79] Traditional Chinese doctors seek to facilitate Qi energy flow through the body to treat disease, disharmony, and imbalance. Traditionally, Qi in the body is sometimes compared to water. That is, it wants to flow toward balance. Optimum health occurs, according to both Traditional Chinese Medicine and Tai Chi, when the Qi flows smoothly throughout the body. Likewise, damage is caused when Qi flow is blocked or weakened. One's personal Qi can be clouded or affected by a variety of factors including intrusive thoughts and emotions, feelings, activities, food, one's environment, and so on. Having said all of that, there is nothing magical about Qi, as Sifu has said many times. The body is comprised of bioelectric "circuits" and

---

79 Yang, Jwing Ming, 1997. Kaptchuk, 1986.

presents a bioelectric field. Organs such as the heart, brain, and the like, emit their own smaller, self-similar fields. Each individual cell emits its own smaller, self-similar field, as well.[80] We can measure these fields fairly easily, and we can measure variations in each field that occur when we are engaged in different activities. Western medical science has yet to find evidence that meridians or reservoirs are physical organs. However, bioelectrical energy in the body is demonstrably measurable. This is Qi, Sifu says. It can be cultivated and enhanced.

---

80 Yang, 1989, suggests that different types of cells offer varying levels of conductivity and resistance. Fat cells, for example offer more electrical resistance. It is likely that the fibrous, inelastic fascia cells do as well. On the other hand, nerve cells, neurons in the brain, and similar, are likely to be highly conductive. As I explained in an earlier chapter, I have a hypothesis that patterns of cell conductivity and resistance throughout the body shape and form the Qi energy meridians throughout the body.

Chapter 13: **Jin or Jing**

Of the five energies, this is the one I have less to say about at the present time. For now, it is enough to say that Jin is the expression or emission of energy. Remember how we talked about how feelings become named into emotions and emotions are forms of expression? Similarly, Jin is the expression of energy translated from Qi. Think about it this way: We can compare Jin to the work of the engine. The engine of your car, for example, is what makes the car move. In a mechanical or engineering sense, the work of an engine might be to move a load or create some change in the world at large. The fuel represents Qi and the work of the engine is Jin.

With respect to Jin, there are many different forms this expression might take. The many forms of Jin are differentiated by their function, by the work they do. For example, suppose you wish to connect with the person standing in front of you. Do you want to tickle them? That takes a particular kind of energy or a particular type of touch. Do you wish to caress them? That requires a similar but distinct energy. Maybe you wish to strike them. That strike could be a push. It could be a percussive punch or slap intended to cause pain. It could be a strike that is meant to disrupt internal energy pathways, or it could be a touch that restores the flow of internal energy and heals or helps a person. Maybe you are sparring and wish to land an authentic strike, but you don't want to hurt your training partner and so you aim to impact only the fabric of their shirt. All of these and many more are variations of expressing energy. All of these connections are powered by intention, imagination, focus, and sensing your opponent. Essentially, if our intent is to launch a strike, throw a punch, or similar, we can use a cultivated sense of Jin to make that strike more powerful and to direct the shape and function of the energy at impact.

There are two things you should know about cultivating and developing Jin energy. First, if you choose to walk down the path of understanding and developing your Jin, understand that it will be a long journey. Expect it to take years of study. Be patient. Second, understand that you are taking on a great responsibility. This represents a deep, distant corner of the Tai Chi world, one that many teachers are unable or perhaps unwilling to explain in any detail. It represents a great responsibility to hand to a student. If misused or misunderstood, the application of Jin energy can cause great damage. If this is something that interests you, I recommend that you find a knowledgeable teacher who can guide you.

There is a difference between the expression of energy and the expression of ego. With respect to creativity, for example, we can suggest that the impulse to be creative — that energetic fire — represents one aspect of Jin. That is, if you are the sort of person who enjoys any sort of creative pursuit, the pursuit itself might be considered Jin. Jin is also doing any sort of work in the sense of affecting something in the world around you or expressing any sort of energy, perhaps for the sake of exercise. The idea of cultivating Jin is to make the energy use more efficient — for example, using the same amount of energy to do more work.

Lastly, at the beginning of the book, we talked about the idea of Kung Fu as applying to any sort of effort or endeavor that requires practice, patience, or presence of mind. In a philosophical sense, cultivating Jin is analogous to purifying your intent or purpose in what might be otherwise thought of as an ordinary or mundane activity so that your efforts are more efficient and effective. In other words, the cultivation or development of Jin might characterize or color any activity in which one needs to be reminded that the effort itself is the purpose instead of chasing the result.

Chapter 14: Spirit

Wuji

"He who fights with monsters should look to himself that he does not become the monster. And if you gaze into the abyss long enough, the abyss gazes into you"[81]

Or this:

He who excels in combat does not let himself be roused. That the warriors of old ... came to learn how to apply the secret of emptiness; How to ensure that the enemy's sword, though aimed at flesh encounters void; And how to destroy the foe by striking with dispassion. Hatred arouses wrath; wrath breeds excitement; excitement leads to carelessness which, to a warrior, brings death.... A swordsman or an archer's aim is scariest when his mind concentrated on the work in hand and is indifferent to failure or success... Stillness in the heart of movement is the secret to power"[82].

Sifu says, "First, find your balance. Then move." You can throw yourself into the Abyss or into the Void.

Choose. We talked about functional balance just a moment ago and how it relates to the body and to moving. Let's look at the balance as it relates to the spirit. We begin this part with deep thoughts. Deep thoughts, indeed.

---

81   Friedrich Nietzsche

82   Liu and Bracy, Ba Gua: Hidden Knowledge in the Taoist Internal Martial Art, 1998, p. 36.

The Abyss

Nietzsche's Abyss versus the Void, called Wuji by the Daoists: They are completely different things. The dictionary says they both denote vast emptiness and it may be suggested that they sound like the same thing. However, they are not.

The Abyss is a deep, dark hole. It is the darkness, a lack of light or hope. It is the black of night. The Abyss is despair. The Abyss is what happens when we are consumed by emotions: sadness, fear, anger, and so on. The Abyss is drowning ourselves in our victim's story. The corrosive effect of unbalanced emotions, intrusive thoughts, or ruminations also begin to weigh on one's sense of self. They begin to affect how we move through the world. In other words, an unbalanced mind over time erodes and corrodes the spirit. Anxiety, depression, grief, anger, compulsive or obsessive love, lust — we might think of them as deadly sins. Instead, think of them as traps of the spirit. Instead of worrying about atoning for them, seek to find your way out of the traps. As Nietzsche suggested, if you let it, the Abyss will teach you to become the thing you wish to fight. Or else, connect to a higher power beyond yourself, find your elevated spirit, become a more spiritually developed person.

The Void

The Void, on the other hand, is stillness. Focus. Calm. Land of no thought. It is the stillness before action. It is the letting go of ego, self-concern, and tension. The Void is the Song that connects us to the Cosmos, Source, Spirit, God, however you wish to describe it. The Void is the imperative to protect ourselves and the people we love while letting go of the ego and letting go of attachments to the outcome. Letting go of ego and attachments in the service of self-defense may seem counterintuitive. However, while letting go of ego, we grow in intention and wisdom. We come to discover that we are connected to our opponent. We fight them both viciously and with great compassion, as though we care a great deal about them. At least. That is Tai Chi. That is what Sifu says.

The Void means cutting with your sword in the moment. Cut with precision and without hesitation. The Void represents the recognition and dismissal of noise, ego. The Void wants to teach us to listen, to hear that that everything is connected. Focus. The Void is the recognition and dismissal of noise; ego. The Void wants to teach you that all things are connected. The Void is true focus. True connection. These moments teach us the difference between Void and the Abyss.

Sifu says, "First, find your balance. Then move."

Calm. Cut.

You can throw yourself into the Abyss or into the Void.

On a More Prosaic Level

Wow. We have just done quite a lot of heavy spiritual lifting. Take a breath.

Now. On a more prosaic level, spirit might be said to represent personal agency, effectiveness, the ability to exert oneself in a way that matters or makes a difference. It represents the understanding and cultivation of Jin.

This is not the same thing as reaching for a goal. Reaching for a goal is situational. If we reach for one goal and meet it, we congratulate ourselves and move onto the next one. For example, completing this book is a goal I have had. We need goals. That is how things get done. However, if we engage with the Great Taiji or seek wisdom and understanding simply for the love of doing so or to make ourself a better person, there is no specific or definitive goal. There is only gaining in wisdom. Personal spirit represents your stance or mindset in reaching for that goal. It relates to a person's disposition or presentation or personality. It relates to a person's agency.

When we speak about agency, we are talking about an individual's ability to feel self-effective in the work they choose or value most, their relationships, or their self-realized missions and meaning. How effective do you feel you are in your career or your relationships? How stuck do you feel? How heard do you feel in your relationships? Maybe you don't feel heard. Maybe you feel ignored or misunderstood. Those are aspects of agency or spirit.

Agency might also describe how connected you feel to yourself, to Earthly energy, or to your community. How connected do you feel to heavenly energies? This could be God, your ancestors, the Cosmos, or whatever you chose to call it. Maybe to you, it's Universal energy or simply Spirit. How do you present energetically? How invested are you in your comparison to others or in the acquisition of shiny objects? These suggest something about Spirit, too. How devoted are you to reaching for contentment with your life or with your self?

The study of martial arts in general and Tai Chi in particular is the study of agency. When we talk about self-defense, we talk about our physical self — or on a more philosophical level, we want to preserve our ego. We want to avoid blows to fragile ego. When it comes to martial arts, however, we are studying how to impose our will on the world. Issues of morality or authority aside, we are learning how to become effective or competitive or victorious. We are learning agency. The question becomes whether we are doing this for the advancement of our ego or in service to our community. Sifu often describes being a servant samurai. By this he means to create a flavor of agency based on melding service to the community with a devotion to ideals and values that are higher than one's self.

From the perspective of spirit, Tai Chi requires first self-discipline and self-development. It teaches us to become aware of ourselves, then others, then the environment. It teaches us to sense and to cultivate Qi energy and then express it as Jin. Hopefully, this is applied to service to others, patience, compassion, and so on. Tai Chi practice has a way of bending one's experience toward both the internal mind and the external environment but away from the self. This is what we mean by getting oneself out of one's head or getting out of one's way.

Agency is like water. Sometimes it is calm. Sometimes it flows. The greater the pressure, the faster it wears away at the rock. However, even a slow drip can erode a stone. Yes, the speed at which the rock erodes depends on the water pressure, and from this, we might be tempted to apply more pressure and speed up the process. However, moving with patience and certainty is an acceptable strategy.

Wisdom stories from various traditions often speak about enlightenment as some sort of destination or completion. The end of the journey or race. However, I imagine that if you were to ask an enlightened person, they would tell you that the journey toward understanding and wisdom never really ends. Buddhists might say that the Buddha's journey as someone who liberated himself from the cycle of Samsara – birth, death and rebirth – comes to a welcome end at their last earthly breath. Maybe, even that is not the last conclusion.

Tai Chi wants to teach us that if you must fight, fight viciously. Win without guilt, but do so with the mind of compassion for your opponent. Sifu offers this wisdom: Fight effectively. Develop and defend yourself. Elevate the people that you care about. But fight as though your opponent is also someone whom you care about.

With respect to Tai Chi, awareness sometimes requires that someone's attention might at any particular moment be focused on earthly energies or on the Cosmos. I think this is one meaning of the Taiji, the Yin Yang symbol. It represents the interplay of earthly Qi and heavenly Qi. A person is an agent with two poles, like a magnet with one energetic pole firmly affixed to Earth and one pointed to the sky, the Cosmos.

And So

In a moment of confrontation, depression, anxiety, or stress; in a moment of unbalance, listen. Feel the righteousness of your ego and your anger. Feel your feelings. Feel the watchful gaze of your teacher. Feel your intention. Find your center. Find your breath. Feel the breeze on your face. Feel your clothes; The fabric of your sleeve on your arm. Find the tremble in your hand or the smooth surface of the table. Feel the floor through your feet. Find your distal pulse or the Point of Bubbling Qi in your feet. Find your opponent. Where does he stand? Find his center. Feel his energy and his intention. Watch him move. Get there first. Which of all of these is more beautiful? Which of these is noise? This is awareness. This is Wuji. Stillness. Now move. This is Tai Chi.

Chapter 15: The Lantern Is Lit

The lantern is lit. It casts a bright glow on the steps ahead. Beyond that, the future is always shadowed in mystery. We cannot see too far down the path. What does it mean that we know our final destination but we can not see it?

At breakfast one morning, Sifu asked this: "Suppose you knew that you would die tomorrow at 2 p.m. If there is anything that you still wanted to do or say… If your final day is a crashing attempt to finish unfinished business, then you have been doing it wrong."

I think that what he meant by that is that we should be spending every day doing and saying what we need to do and say so that we can greet the end satisfied and with calmness and dignity and perhaps with a sense of wonder and awe.

Meanwhile, if you seek enlightenment, first do the dishes.

I don't recall where that slogan came from. Perhaps, it's Buddhist. Maybe it's a paraphrase of something the rabbis said. It suggests a sort of struggle between the daily process of life and seeking wisdom. It speaks to me because sometimes I do have dishes stacked in the sink. My house is sometimes untidy. It can be cluttered: There are books everywhere and notebooks and tchotchkes and knickknacks, curiosities, and so on. And my cat. It might be said that untidiness or clutter is a form of noise. Distraction. Perhaps it is. Clutter might also be a form of familiarity: Objects that hold meaning and memories of happy times may be comforting spirits. At least until there is an avalanche on my desk and I am literally or metaphorically buried by clutter. Perhaps.

It might also be said that everything I own also owns a piece of me. In other words, there is a materialistic relationship between me and my possessions. I worry about my property, my stuff. What if someone robs me? Or steals one of my books? What if there's a fire, and I lose everything? What if I do lose everything? How much time and energy need I devote to worrying about my stuff? How much of that is noise?

When I am focused on Tai Chi practice, even those thoughts represent noise. On the other hand, if I am so compulsive that my house must be clean before I practice Tai Chi, that is noise too. And if I am cleaning all the time, when do I have time to practice? Balance in all things.

I am not a Buddhist. Though, it's quite a grand thing to aspire to the spiritual heights of personal enlightenment. For others, the pinnacle of personal development might be mastery of a musical instrument or mastery of Tai Chi or another discipline. We respect authentic seekers a great deal. However we typically only recognize them when they reach the summit. In case you haven't yet figured it out, with respect to Tai Chi there is no summit. Only more peaks to climb, each taller yet. With respect to seekers, we don't often see the effort that goes into their ascent. We don't often recognize the work they have done or the challenges of their climb. We don't see that part. That work? That is Kung Fu. That is Tai Chi.

For me? I do have to keep at least one foot firmly planted on the soil of terra mundane – the ordinary things like dishes in the sink or daily scraping for my coin. I suspect that I am not alone in this. Not everyone can become enlightened. Buddha. Somebody has to cook the rice. Not everyone can or should spend their entire days meditating under the Bodhi tree or sitting in a cave deciphering shadows on the wall. Somebody has to pour the coffee. Somebody has to file the tax returns. Somebody has to turn the proverbial crank that makes the world go around. Somebody has to keep the lights on, so to speak. We have to do all of these tasks so that we can have moments to practice faithfully. There must be balance.

At the same time, not every one has to be Buddha. We already have the Sermon of the Flower, for example. There is much still to learn from it, but there is no reason to rewrite it. The good news is this: now that we have it, anyone can choose to take a moment to "read" that sermon.

Maybe the age of masters is fading because in many respects, we've already discovered all that stuff. Add to that, life is becoming ever more complicated, and frankly, added complexity is disruptive. Perhaps it is difficult to balance the pursuit of self-development with the demands of everyday life: work, family, and so on. But hasn't that always been the problem? In today's world, we also have far more time-management technology, and we seem to have plenty of leisure or personal time, or at least more so than in ages past. We also seem to have plenty of distractions to manage as well.

Not everyone can throw away all their ordinary cares and daily chores. Not everyone can "go all Cheng San Feng," play hermit, and hide away in a cave for years to meditate—even if, some people might think that sounds like fun. Not everyone has the time or the will to perfect their understanding of the art of their choosing, Tai Chi. At some point, we must also engage with the world. There are choices to be made about how we spend our time.

Happily, we really don't need to reinvent the wheel. With respect to Tai Chi, understanding of the art grows every day. We can learn from those who came before us. We've already had our Cheng San Feng, our Yang Chen Fu, and others whose past teachings light the path ahead. I can learn more quickly and can reach greater depths of understanding because the teachers who came before have lit the way forward. The lantern is lit, and it shows us the way.

Maybe the lantern glows brightest just before the dim. Maybe the age of the great masters has faded because every day there is ever more information available about every master who ever walked. Maybe all of the great discoveries with respect to Tai Chi have already been made. Maybe all of the mysteries have been clearly discussed.

(We are coming to the end of this book, after all.) We certainly don't have to search as hard to prise out secrets because those who came before us have passed along their wisdom. Today, we have apps, and we have YouTube. Everything is on YouTube.

How would my Teacher compare to Yang Lu Chan? How would your teacher? Who can rightly say. Does it even matter? Sifu has an advantage over every master who has come before him. He has access to their wisdom and insights. He has read their books and studied the teachings they have passed down. In a metaphorical or even metaphysical sense, my teacher is the avatar of every master who has come before him. Your teacher might be, too — but only if they seek to be. And only if they hold on to the stories and traditions and if they have students to pass along their wisdom.

Seriously, I don't believe that the age of masters has passed us by. At the same time, I also don't believe that you can throw a crusty shoe and hit some guy on the street corner who happens to be a Tai Chi master. There might not be enough masters to put one in every Starbucks or on every street corner. (Except on YouTube: Everyone on YouTube is a master.) True masters should be difficult to come by. They should be sought out, prized, revered, and not disposable. If you choose to stop training with one, it should come at a cost. The costs of achievement should be set high. By costs of achievement, I don't mean monetary expense. I mean costs in terms of time and dedication. I mean Gong Fu. And certainly, any master worth their salt would certainly know enough to duck your thrown shoe.

The Book of Changes, Part II

August 2019: We were at Sifu's house in suburban Cincinnati. It was a yellow two-story Cape Cod. On Saturday mornings, we would gather in his living room for class. Now we were helping him move out. He had been renting the house, and the landlord had decided to sell. Sifu had to leave. A bunch of us from the Tai Chi community were helping him to move out...and downsize.

Renovations had just begun at the Powder Factory. The dilapidated manufacturing complex had been sold, and plans had been made to repurpose it the into a community of apartments, condominiums, and a micro-brewery. While the rebuilding was going on, Sifu was eager return. He was happy to move into a construction trailer on the property. It was a temporary fix. When the renovations were complete, he would be offered an apartment, and he wanted to keep his foot in the door.

Construction trailers do not come with a whole lot of space, so he had to downsize. He had a lifetime collection of martial arts objects he had to let go of: books, training gear, and so on. Attachments. Impermanence. I watched him hand a big binder to one of his senior students. It was one of those three-ring binders, and it was stuffed with pages. It was his personal book of teaching notes. I recall thinking that I would have loved to have gotten a peek at the treasures in those pages. The book of collected wisdom. That moment had a lot of significance for me. And I'm sure it did for that particular senior student as well. To me, it represented the passing of the torch from master to senior student. There was an element of finiteness, a recognition of mortality. The passing of the torch. It reminded me of how much I wanted to still learn from Sifu, and that the clock was ticking.

A thinking man's personal book of thoughts, insights, and wisdom. A collection from decades of practice. It was the transmission of ideas and understanding to the next generation. To me, passing along that work suggested a sense of mortality – change. I could suggest that along the journey, we shouldn't fear change. Somehow, we do.

Impermanence

Sifu said in class yesterday that Tai Chi is the study of change. Like many things he says, I believe he meant several different things all at once. For one thing, Tai Chi changes how we are. It helps us become ourselves. It helps us move. The poses become moves. The moves become techniques for self-defense, and the techniques eventually become self-expression. This is the point at which the traditions become art. This is the point at which we stop reacting to impulse and begin to become curious.

Think of it this way. Imagine that you get into a conflict, and you've been practicing your forms diligently. You've gotten good enough to ward off anything your opponent throws at you. Any argument, strike, punch, kick, and so on, that he throws at you, you can answer. If you get to this point, you would be a formidable fighter, indeed. What would that be like for you? How would that skill change the way you walk through the world? Would you still experience fear or anxiety in conflicts? Would they be the same fears and anxieties you had before? That is one landmark on the road to mastery.

Suppose you continue to train and learn. Eventually you learn to anticipate your opponent. One day, you get into a conflict, and you realize you can anticipate every move your opponent makes. You know your opponent even if you have never encountered him before. You can read his body language. You can read his weightedness. You can read his intent. By anticipating your opponent, you learn a number of valuable lessons. First, you learn to change your move in the moment. You can alter your response on the fly or adapt to changing circumstances. That is another landmark on the road to mastery.

Second, you learn you can actually defend yourself by manipulating your opponent. You can manipulate your opponent's body in one direction or another based on what you do and what kind of energy you put into your moves. Make him step this way or lean that way. Take his balance and structure. Suddenly, you learn that the only thing that really holds you back is fear. But by then, it's too late: your fear has already vanished. Then, you realize that you have become curious. You have become curious about which techniques work in which situations and how you can apply different patterns. That is Tai Chi.

You also become curious about your opponent: Why is he angry or afraid or confrontational? Once you reach that awareness, suddenly he becomes a real person instead of a cardboard cutout. You become empathetic, and you connect to him is ways you might not otherwise. At this point, what role does your own fear play in the conflict? It gets squeezed out by something else, and something really weird happens. In that instant, you become a much better fighter, and you realize you do not need to fight at all. That is Wuji. That is balance.

But there is more yet. Tai Chi is the study of change. It is transformative. Remember the I Ching? In his book Mastery: the Keys to Success and Long-Term Fulfillment, George Leonard writes, "To learn is to change. Education, whether it involves books, body or behavior, is a process that changes the learner."[83] This is one of the grand treasures of Tai Chi. The art wants to help us change, transform, into the best versions of ourself. What ever that might look like for us. And it helps us adapt to changing circumstances. As we grow and mature, our bodies change. As we gain in wisdom and understanding, our thinking changes (hopefully). Furthermore, our world changes dramatically as we move through it, almost with every step. Ideally, we want to adapt in order to better meet changes in our life. Awareness the initial step in the process of adaptation.

Then

I think that if you asked him, Sifu would tell you that his treasures are the relationships he has with loyal students and his lifelong accumulation of wisdom and knowledge. There is nothing else you can take with you.

Any true trove of wisdom will eventually come to the understanding that every life is finite. Impermanence is the hallmark of the human condition. Mortality. So we come to the question of what to do with the wisdom we've accumulated in the face of our own

---

83   Leonard, Mastery, p. 118.

mortality. The prevailing wisdom in the West is that we get precisely one life — one chance. And there is no evidence — no discussion — that you can take any of your "wealth" with you. By wealth, of course, I mean wealth, any objects you treasure or aspects of your ego. It's sort of nihilistic in a way. Imagine being on your death bed, surrounded by a pile of things — tchotchkes, mementos, or trinkets that have meaning or value for you. Anything of sentimental, or worse, material value. You can transmit your wealth to your progeny, and you can transmit wisdom to your students.

For example, Sifu owns an antique sword that he swears he has wielded in a past life. It is certainly an antique, at least several hundreds of years old. The sword has an weird kind of energy to it. It feels as though it has history, as though it has tasted blood. Sifu has traced its age by its blade design to a particular time and place in ancient Japan when such blade designs were fashionable.

I am reminded of Chen's saber. The Chen family still claims to possess it after many generations. Some objects accumulate a particular energy over the ages of history. Wealth, wisdom and personal tokens have a way being passed along to future generations. Objects can have that sense of permanence. And the transmission of understanding occurs through family lore, books, and students.

Immortality

There are stories. But really, who knows if they are true. Immortality. It's an interesting idea, of course. The Daoist alchemists seem to be very interested in uncovering the secrets of extended life. For them, immortality represents the pinnacle of achievement. Transformation. The Buddhists, on the other hand, are more interested in freeing themselves from the nearly endless cycle of reincarnation: birth, death, and rebirth. Of course, other religions have their own ideas and beliefs about life, death, and what comes after. And while some of these may be more familiar to Western readers, Tai Chi finds its roots in in Daoist and Buddhist philosophies. While Tai Chi is in no way a religion and does not interfere with whatever religious beliefs a person may or may not hold dear, it does offer clues for those who are willing to consider them for connecting to the universe, or to God, or whatever you prefer to call the great Taiji.

Set aside questions of spirituality for a moment. Immortality. The word means everlasting life. Or perhaps, it means simply life extended beyond the normal range of years. Of course, the normal range of years available to a person is only an average, and there will always be outliers on either end of that. There will always be those who live long and those whose lives are cut short. There are always stories about someone's cranky old grandmother or grandfather who smoked, swore, and drank everyday and lived to a grand old age. Perhaps. Did they live a life of balance?

What I offer you is the possibility that Tai Chi, and by extension Qi Gong, may offer something of an extended life. Tai Chi and Qi Gong do have reputations, well-earned perhaps, for warding off the ravages of time and age and promoting vitality and well-being. Both arts promote being active longer, more flexible, more supple into old age. They may add to the number of years we might live. What if they could make the number of years we do live better? What if Tai Chi could help us avoid the kind of long, slow, painful decline that afflicts so many toward the end of their lives? What if it could help keep us vital and vigorous? Would that not strike the people around us as a kind of immortality?

Something else to think about. What if immortal is not an adjective but a noun, a word synonymous with sage or wise person. It might not be too far a stretch to suppose that in ages past, when normal life expectancy was short, anyone old was presumed to also be wise. Maybe they possessed some secret of health and longevity. Maybe they only appeared to be immortal because they retained their vigor and vitality while people around them declined and dropped off much sooner. That might be one way to look at it. Still, it's hard to completely let go of the romantic image of a spirit like Cheng San Feng prowling around the Wudang Mountains for hundreds of years.

What about this. What if we could rid ourselves of the fear of dying? What would it be like to live life without the fear of life's inevitable end? What if true immortality really means passing along our legacy of wisdom to those who come after us? Maybe Tai Chi has something to say about that too.

The lantern is lit. The path forward is clear...for at least a few steps. After that, it's up to you. Fare forward, Voyager.

Conclusion: The Experience of Frogs

First, a story about eagles.: There is a story about an old Tai Chi master who could speak to animals. There is a story about a conversation he had with an eagle. You see, the eagle was explaining the idea of flying and why he loved it so much.

"You reach out and greet the wind currents. You can float along them through the mountains," the eagle was saying.

"That is just like Tai Chi," the old master replied. "You reach out and greet your opponent — who might be yourself. You greet incoming strikes and float along them."

"But you can't fly in the mountains on cloudy days," the eagle mused. "Sometimes there are rocks in the clouds. If you hit one, it would be bad. You would get hurt."

"Rocks? Yes. Certainly you don't want to get hit," the old master replied. "We study Tai Chi so we might avoid the rocks by clearing away the fog and clouds."

The Experience of Frogs

"People today tend to dissect the frog to understand its body and functions, whereas Zhuangzi [Chang Tzu] wanted to experience the living quality of the frog. Many people like the shape and color of a flower whereas Zhuangzi liked the life of the flower itself."[84]

---

84 Liang and Wu, 1997, p. 79. Zhuangzi was a Chinese philosopher and follower of Lao-tzu. Zhaungzi wrote a book referred to as "Zhuangzi" or "Chung Ztu." Lao-tzu is the author of the Dao Te Ching, The Way of the Dao.

WESTERN MEDICAL SCIENCE

Western medical science has long enjoyed the practice of dissecting things — frogs, for example — in the pursuit of better understanding of how they work. Western medicine has become very good at examining the pieces and parts and understanding how they fit together. As a result, we have learned quite a lot about the muscular system, the organs, and the attending ligaments and tendons. We understand the cardiovascular system, the circulation of the blood, and the nervous system. We can even create models of the brain that indicate which parts are active during various mental, physical, and emotional events. We understand that the body is a collection of interrelated parts and systems.

In Western medicine, when a patient comes in with a problem, something is wrong. Something doesn't work right. Something hurts. The doctor looks for signs and symptoms of discomfort, dysfunction, and disease. From there, they determine a diagnosis by which they seek to return the patient to comfort or base-line functioning. The doctor might prescribe medical procedure, therapy, or medicine. It is a very mechanistic and a somewhat reductionist process. In other words, there is a broken or worn-out part, and it gets repaired or replaced. There is dysfunction, discomfort, or disease, and the doctor aims to fix or replace the offending mechanism or eliminate the cause of it.

CHINESE MEDICAL PHILOSOPHY

By contrast, according to the Chinese medical paradigm, the patient presenting with a complaint is thought to be off balance: "Why is there disharmony?"[85] Traditional Chinese Medicine seeks to restore the patient to wholistic balance. It might do this by asking not only about the source of each symptom and sign of dis-ease or dis-function, but how do all of the symptoms and signs fit together. It might also ask what is going on in the patient's life or environment

---

85   Kaptchuk, p. 116.

that might be causing unbalance. And while each symptom becomes a clue, the idea is not to reduce the symptom, dis-ease or dysfunction individually. The idea is to seek the underlying cause – even if it is external – and treat the patient's experience. The idea is to seek balance.

THE POINT

Western medical science has a lot to teach us. It is a powerful method of understanding complex systems. We examine each part or section in great detail and test it to learn its properties. There is the implicit understanding that each piece or part is also part of the whole; that by understanding the parts, we can draw a picture of the whole. So, yes. We might dissect frogs but doing so is in service of better understanding frogs and how they work. However, doing so also comes with one attendant problem: Once you dissect a frog, you can no longer enjoy the experience of watching it be a frog.

We have spent quite a lot of time talking about the various pieces and parts of Tai Chi. We have pulled the art apart and examined each component part or aspect, one by one. And that is exactly how we have to do it. Every single piece is meant to be a conversation and a practice. We discuss, test, and play with each principle, concept, or detail of movement one by one. Slowly, we adapt them into our understanding. The idea, of course, is to put the whole thing back together again once we understand the parts.

FROGS AND TAI CHI

There is another way to think about the way we experience frogs. Yes. Of course, they are bulbous and bumpy and slimy and squishy. What if we could simply find pleasure in our experience of them? What if we could simply admire them for their peculiar beauty and character? What if we could spend a moment thinking about what it might be like to be a frog?

Frogs are very adaptable. They do one thing really well. They know how to be frogs. Frogs are the best creatures on the planet at doing frog things. They catch and eat bugs and flies. They keep themselves warm in the winter. They begin life as tadpoles and transform into the form of their greatest potential. That form is magnificent in a frog sort of way. It a matter of survival — learning how to adapt to their environment. However, I can't imagine that they spend a lot of time wishing they could be something else.

We can dissect frogs in order to better understand their mechanism and functioning. We can do the same for Tai Chi. The advantage that Tai Chi has over dissecting frogs is that at some point, we can (should) stop thinking about the details. We should stop thinking about whether we are doing it right and simply enjoy the experience of Tai Chi. Frogs never stop to think about how to be a frog. Perhaps, at the end of the day, Tai Chi wants to teach us how to fulfill the biological imperative of becoming our whole self without doubt or hesitation. What if I could learn to simply be like the frog?

That is Wuji.

One Last Note

Scott Rodell is an internationally respected Tai Chi teacher and historian who specializes in Qing Dynasty swords. In his book Taiji Notebook for Martial Artists: Essays by a Yang Family Taijiquan Practitioner, Rodell asks a question which I find inspiring. I like to think of it as one of the Great Ultimate Questions, and as such, it is well worth repeating here. Rodell wonders: If you encountered a true Tai Chi master and could ask any one, single question — about anything — what would you ask?

You only get one question. Anything at all. What would you want to know? Rodell's answer is elegant, simple, and profound.

He would ask this: What time does class start?

References

Bisio, Tom. Xing Yi Quan: Art of Inner Transformation. Outskirts Press, 2019.

Chan, Wing-tsit, trans. A Sourcebook in Chinese Philosophy. Princeton University Press, 1963.

Cheng, Man-Ch'ing. Cheng Tzu's Thirteen Treatises on T'ai Chi Ch'uan. Translated by Benjamin Pang Jeng Lo and Martin Inn. Blue Snake Books, 1985.

Cheng, Man-Ch'ing. Master Cheng's New Method of Tai Chi Self-Cultivation. Translated by Mark Hennessy, Blue Snake Books, 1999.

Clark, Bernie. YinSights: A Journey into the Philosophy & Practice of Yin Yoga. B. Clark, 2007.

Cleary, Thomas, translator. The Taoist I Ching . Shambhala Classics, 1986.

Da, Liu. T'ai Chi Ch'uan and Meditation. Schocken Books, 1991.

Daly, M. The Heart Treasure of Taijiquan. Purple Cloud Press, 2021.

Diepersloot, Jan. The Tao of Yiquan: The Method of Awareness in the Martial Arts, Volume 2 of the Warriors of Stillness Trilogy. Walnut Creek, California. Center for Healing and the Arts, 1999.

Doidge, Norman, MD. The Brain's Way of Healing: Remarkable Discoveries and Recoveries from the Frontiers of Neuroplasticity. Brunswick, Victoria: Scribe, 2017.

Dunning, Jennifer. "Sophia Delza Glassgold, 92, Dancer and Teacher." The New York Times, 7 July 1996.

Hanson, Rick, and Richard Mendius. Buddha's Brain: The Practical Neuroscience of Happiness, Love, and Wisdom. New Harbinger Publications, 2009.

Huang, Alfred. Complete Tai-Chi: The Definitive Guide to Physical and Emotional Self-Development. Charles E. Tuttle, Co., 1993.

Hughart, Barry. The Bridge of Birds: A Novel of an Ancient China that never was. Ballantine, 1985.

Humphreys, Christmas. Concentration and Meditation: A Manual of Mind Development. Element Books, 1987.

Isaacson, Walter. Einstein: His Life and Universe. Simon and Schuster, 2007.

Jou, Tsung Hwa. The Tao of Tai-Chi Chuan: Way to Rejuvenation. Edited by Shoshana Shapiro. Tai Chi Foundation, 1991.

Jung, Carl G. Man and His Symbols. Dell Publishing, 1968.

Kabat-Zinn, Jon. Full Catastrophe Living: Using the Wisdom of Your Body and Mind to Face Stress, Pain, and Illness. Bantam Books, 2013

Kaptchuck, Ted J. Chinese Medicine: The Web That Has No Weaver. Rider and Company, 1986.

Katchmer, George A. The Tao of BioEnergetics: East and West. Yang's Martial Arts Association, 1993.

Kelly, Dave. "How an American Dancer Introduced Tai Chi to America." SMA Bloggers, 23 Sept. 2015, https://smabloggers.com. Accessed 4 Aug. 2021.

Lee, Bruce. John Little, ed. The Tao of Gung Fu: Commentaries on the Chinese Martial Arts. Clarendon, VT: Tuttle, 2016.

Leonard, George. Mastery: The Keys to Success and Long-Term Fulfillment. Penguin Books, 1991.

Lewis, Dennis. The Tao of Natural Breathing for Health, Well-Being and Inner Growth. Mountain Wind Publishing, 1997.

Liang, Shou-Yu, and Weng Ching Wu. Qigong Empowerment: Guide to Medical, Taoist, Buddhist, Wushu Energy Cultivation. Way of the Dragon Publishing, 1997.

Liang, Shou-Yu, and Weng Ching Wu. Tai Chi Chuan: 24 and 48 Postures with Martial Applications. D. Breiter-Wu, Ed. YMAA Publication Center, 1996.

Liang, Shou-Yu, J.-M. Yang, and Weng Ching Wu. Baguazhang (Emei Baguazhang): Chinese Internal Martial Arts; Theory and Applications. YMAA Publication Center, 1994.

Liao, Waysun. T'ai Chi Classics: New Translations of Three Essential Texts of T'ai Chi Ch'uan with Commentary and Practical Instruction. Shambala Publications, Inc. 1990.

Liu, Hsing-han, and John Bracy. Ba Gua: Hidden Knowledge in the Taoist Internal Martial Art. North Atlantic Books, 1998.

Lowenthal, Wolfe. There Are No Secrets: Professor Cheng Man-ch'ing and his Tai Chi Chuan. Blue Snake Books, 1991.

Opie, James. "The Hunters, the Hunted." Parabola: Tradition, Myth, and the Search for Meaning, 2007.

Rodell, Scott M. Taiji Notebook for Martial Artists: Essays by a Yang Family Taijiquan Practitioner. Seven Stars Books and Video, 1991.

Ronan, Colin A. ed. The Shorter Science and Civilization in China: An Abridgement of Joseph Needham's Original Text. Cambridge University Press, 1978.

Shakespeare, William, The Tragedy of Hamlet, Prince of Denmark. The Folio Society, 1954.

Sophia Delza Papers, Jerome Robbins Dance Division, The New York Public Library for the Performing Arts.

Ueshiba, Morihei. The Art of Peace. Translated by John Stevens. Shambhala, 1992.

Veith, Ilza, trans. The Yellow Emperor's Classic of Internal Medicine. University of California Press, 2002.

Wayne, Peter M., and Mark L. Fuerst. The Harvard Medical School Guide to Tai Chi: Twelve Weeks to a Healthy Body, Strong Heart, and Sharp Mind. Shambhala Publications, Inc., 2013.

Wile, Douglas. Lost T'ai-Chi Classics from the Late Ch'ing Dynasty. State University of New York Press, 1996.

Wile, Douglas. T'ai-Chi's Ancestors: The Making of an Internal Martial Art. Sweet Chi Press, 1999.

Wile, Douglas. Tai-Chi Touchstones: Yang Family Secret Transmissions. Sweet Chi Press, 1983.

Wilhelm, Helmut. The I-Ching, or the Book of Changes. Bollingen Foundation, 1997.

Wilhelm, Helmut and Richard Wilhelm. Understanding the I Ching : The Wilhelm Lectures on the Book of Changes. Princeton University Press, 1995.

Wong, Kiew Kit. The Complete Book of Tai Chi Chuan: A Comprehensive Guide to the Principles and Practice. Cosmos Internet, 2016.

Wright, Simone. First Intelligence: Using the Science and Spirit of Intuition. New World Library, 2014.

Yang, Chengfu. The Essence and Applications of Taijiquan. North Atlantic Books, 2005.

Yang, Dr. Jwing-Ming. Advanced Yang Style Tai Chi Chuan, Volume One: Tai Chi Theory and Tai Chi Jing. YMAA Publication Center, 1987.

Yang, Dr. Jwing-Ming. The Root of Chinese Qigong: Secrets for Health, Longevity, and Enlightenment. YMAA Publication Center, 1997.

Yang, Dr. Jwing-Ming. Qigong: The Secret of Youth: Da Mo's Muscle/Tendon Changing and Marrow/Brain Washing Techniques. Wolfeboro, NH: YMAA Publication, 2000.

Yang, Dr. Jwing-Ming. Taijiquan, Classical Yang Style: The Complete Form and Qigong. Boston: YMAA Publication Center, 1999.

About the Author

Brian L. Meyers

Brian L Meyers has been studying Tai Chi for many years. In addition, he has studied other martial arts including Shotokan Karate, Kempo, and Aikido. He has a 200-hour RYT in Yin, or Taoist Yoga. He received his bachelor's degree from Brandeis University in literature and philosophy, and a master's degree in professional writing and editing from the University of Cincinnati. He is currently working on a master's degree in philosophy, consciousness, and cosmology at California Institute of Integral Studies.

Meyers is also a well sought-out life coach and writing coach. He got his coaching certification from IPEC. He specializes in working with clients who want to understand better writing habits and how to speak to themselves better. He has been helping people get to where they want to be for many years.

He is a proud graduate of Boulder Outdoor Survival School and the National Outdoor Leadership School. He lives in Cincinnati, Ohio.

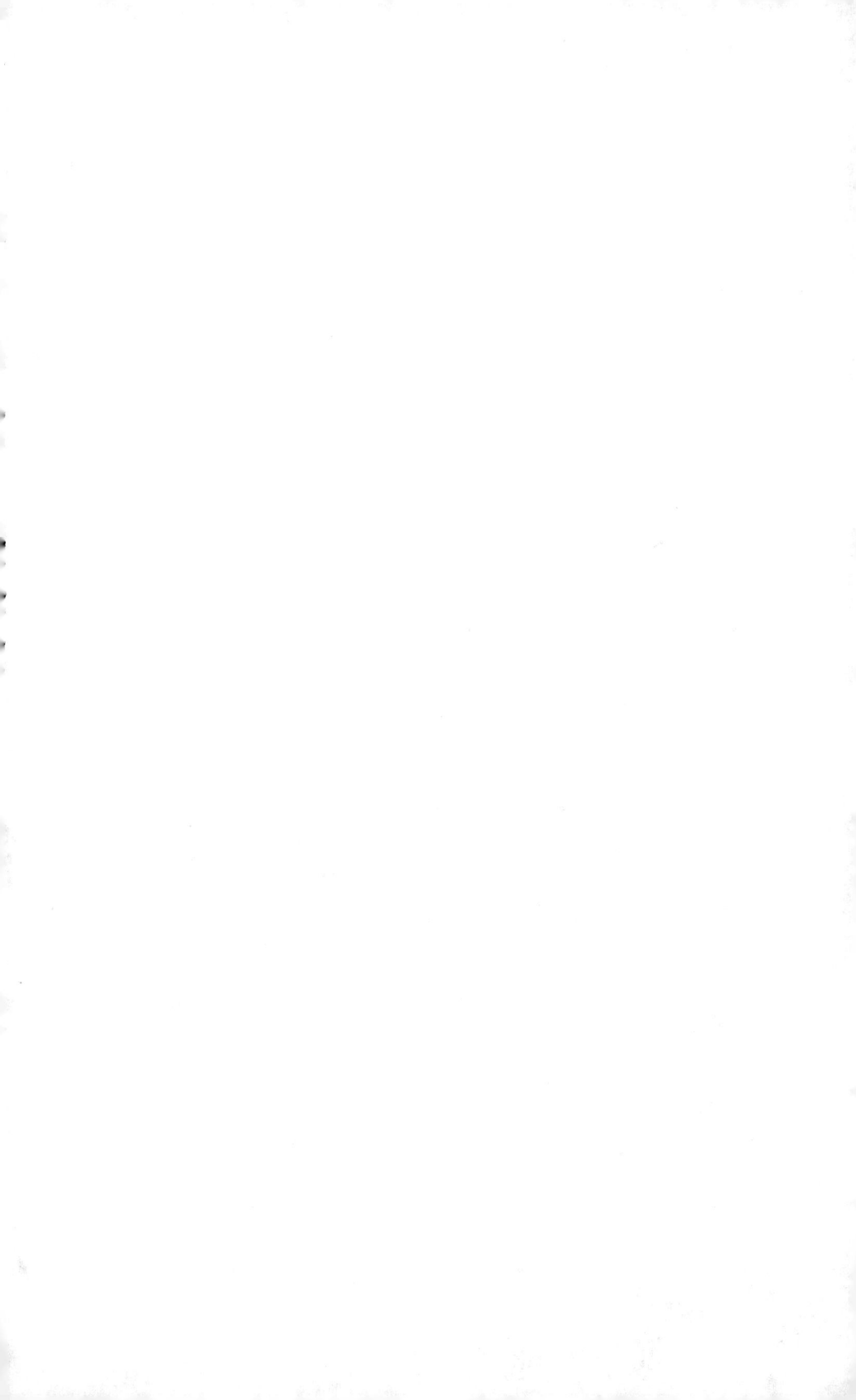

www.ingramcontent.com/pod-product-compliance
Lightning Source LLC
Chambersburg PA
CBHW062220270326
41930CB00009B/1800